The Stress Code

To Isaac who is my inspiration and
Gaby who is my motivation.

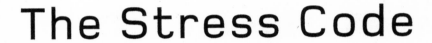

The Stress Code

From Surviving to Thriving
A scientific model for stress resilience

RICHARD SUTTON

MACMILLAN

DISCLAIMER

The information provided in this book is for general informational purposes only.
While we try to keep the information up to date and correct, there are no representations
or warranties, express or implied, about the completeness, accuracy, reliability,
suitability or availability with respect to the information, products,
services, or related graphics contained in this book for any purpose.
Any use of this information is entirely at your own risk.

First published by Quickfox Publishing in 2018 on behalf of Sutton Health
www.suttonhealth.co.za

This edition published in 2018
by Pan Macmillan South Africa
Private Bag X19, Northlands
Johannesburg, 2116
www.panmacmillan.co.za

ISBN: 978-1-77010-657-4
e-ISBN: 978-1-77010-658-1

Copy editing by Pam Thornley
Proofreading by Jane Bowman
Design and typesetting by Triple M Design, Johannesburg
Illustrations by Tina Nel
Cover design by publicide

Printed by **novus print**, a Novus Holdings company

CONTENTS

PREFACE

Stress has always intrigued me. Why is it that some thrive and others barely survive? Despite my long-time interest and life experiences, writing a book about a subject that is impacting each and every one of us was no easy task. The key motivation to take on such an immense project was to find a practical, working solution to an ever-increasing societal challenge. Although I enjoy research, health and finding solutions, I have to admit that it was my professional experiences and recent observations in my work that thrust me into action.

For nearly two decades, I have been managing complex health and performance issues across a variety of domains. I have worked with elite athletes from around the world, national sports federations, and have even been part of a winning Olympic team. Drawing off this experience I have also consulted to thousands of individuals, leading companies, multinational organisations and senior executives. Whether managing pain, complex health issues, productivity or performance, the essence of my work is potential! Potential not only as individuals, but potential as groups and even within large organisations. To actualise potential, break barriers and transcend the average, you have to be healthy, very healthy – both mentally and physically.

Yet there has been profound change in the global health landscape in the last few years. Complex issues involving the immune, nervous, hormonal and reproductive systems are appearing with alarming frequency and increasing severity. Mental health issues have become more prevalent, to the extent that they are the leading burden on the world economy, and our youth are experiencing ailments typically seen in older populations.

Initially, I suspected poor lifestyle habits as the primary driver in this trend. Yet this in itself is not enough to account for the rising prevalence of health issues as, in many respects, basic lifestyle habits are no worse now than they were several years ago.

So I turned my attention to gaining a better understanding of environmental influences, specifically rising pollution levels in our air, water and food, as well as the dramatic proliferation of electromagnetic fields. However distressing my findings were (individually or collectively), as with lifestyle practices, there were holes in the argument, so clearly there was more to the story.

I thought I needed to look even deeper to connect the dots, but the answer was right in front of me. It was always in front of me. Experiencing early life challenges and spending a decade in professional sport, I was aware of the impact of stress. My health had been jeopardised; athletes would sustain injuries and performances crumbled under the strain of chronic stress. More importantly, every day, every week, every year, individuals, teams and organisations were asking me for stress solutions and management guidance.

Without question, chronic stress was the common denominator across all sectors and groups, and like the global decline in health, it has been steadily on the rise. The book's narrative decodes the reasons for this, as well as why chronic stress is so harmful.

If a food is bad for you, you can cut it out. If an activity hurts, you can change your routine. If you're sensitive to pollution, you can move to a cleaner environment. But stress is a conundrum. Not only is it practically unavoidable, stress is both good and bad for you. Small, appropriately timed doses ignite success, help us overcome challenges and grow; but in excess, stress breaks us down.

Realising this, my solution was never going to be avoidance or 'flaky' interventions, but something far more impactful – knowledge! The knowledge to channel and buffer this immensely powerful physiological experience. So, what sets this book apart is that the central theme is understanding the principles that govern the details. In this way, you become the CEO of your health.

Finally, there are two additional messages that can be distilled from the book.

The first is that the truth is complex. It's not a sound bite. There are no quick fixes, superfoods or super-drinks that can have an appreciable effect in the long term. Every health practice or intervention has a time and place, and forms part of the larger whole.

The second is that anything of consequence that can effect real change takes effort, monumental effort, together with consistency.

After four years of slog and reading thousands of journal articles, the book has reached its destination in your hands. I hope you enjoy and benefit from reading it as much as I have from writing it.

HOW TO USE THIS BOOK

This book offers you one of the most comprehensive and structured insights into buffering the adverse effects of stress to promote resilience and achieve your potential in the face of adversity. It is designed to provide solutions at every point along the stress continuum:

- impending stress
- a stressful event
- persistent stressful conditions
- post-stress multi-system compromise, and
- stress in the workplace.

Impending stress

The anticipation of a challenging or important event can often be a major source of stress in our lives. Whether competing in a tournament, having a performance review at work or even going on a long-awaited date, the impending event can cause sleepless nights, not to mention poor outcomes due to over-arousal and anxiety. For example, you are in the middle of gruelling exams. You have put in the hard work, you know the content and even enjoy the subject, but the actual exam pressure is a major stress to you. Moreover, your track record during exams hasn't been good, despite your sound knowledge of the subject.

Chapter 5 Step 1: Change your Perception of Stress gives you the tools and understanding to cope better under the intense pressure, thereby enabling you to achieve the best possible outcome. These tools and skills can be used in many upcoming high-pressure scenarios, such as public speaking, challenging or confrontational meetings, and on the sports field.

A stressful event

Significant stressful events occur frequently in our personal and professional lives, and can have a profound effect on our physical and mental well-being. For example, you have just started a great new job. Despite the fact that you have wanted the new position for years, the first few weeks are distressing, even bringing back distant memories of your first days at school. The surroundings are unfamiliar; social interactions are strained and awkward. You are unsure of your responsibilities and the expectations of others, self-doubt is running rampant and your days are filled with a sense of being out of control with no apparent end in sight.

Fortunately, there are ways in which you can more rapidly adapt and excel in your new role despite the unfamiliar conditions. The solution lies in *Chapter 6 Step 2: Change your Behaviour.* In this chapter, you'll find out how your interpersonal relationships can counteract the physical and emotional impact on your mental and physical health. Moreover, *Chapter 8 Step 4: Rebuild and Repair* offers valuable tools and many interventions that will help you lower your stress responses, buffer the effects of the stress, and promote greater resilience throughout your entire body.

Persistent stressful conditions

Many of us live under relentless, ongoing stress. Often, this is not caused by a single identifiable element, but by the weight of collective life demands and seemingly endless challenges: financial pressures, family pressures, strained relationships, exhausting all-consuming work projects, daily body pain, colds and flu, a to-do list that gets longer by the day ... all amplified by the fact that there is never enough time. The collective strain and frenetic pace put your stress axis into overdrive, propelling you into a compounded state of physical, emotional and cognitive decline. When the decline becomes unmanageable, the result is complete burnout.

Chapter 7 Step 3: Shut it Down places your finger on the stress 'off button'. The interventions are so effective that they are instantaneously able to promote biological balance and restore optimal functionality across all domains. Moreover, the techniques can be tailored to individual circumstances and lifestyle. Some take as little as a few minutes to incorporate successfully.

Post-stress health issues

Many times in life, we feel at our weakest after rather than during protracted periods of stress. Physical fragility, emotional instability and a measurable cognitive decline are often accompanied by extreme exhaustion and antisocial tendencies. Confused as to why we feel this way since there is no current stress to speak of, we seek medical advice and guidance.

This scenario is all too common and is comprehensively addressed in the book. Firstly, *Chapter 2: The Science of Stress* provides a detailed explanation of the stress processes and the impact they have throughout the many systems of the body. This will give you a deep understanding of your experience as well as the direction you need to take to return to optimal health. More importantly, *Chapter 8 Step 4: Rebuild and Repair* provides the necessary lifestyle interventions to successfully and rapidly address this experience. Nutritional supplements, dietary practices, specific exercise protocols and exposure to certain environments are all designed to target important hormones, neuro-chemicals and proteins that steer the body and mind towards strength and robust integrity.

Stress and corporate leadership

Want to enhance employee engagement, reduce absenteeism and improve productivity? *Chapter 3: Stress in the Workplace* provides cutting-edge insights on what drives stress in the workplace and the significant commercial implications. It also provides policy guidelines on how to positively change your professional landscape. Leaders at all levels within an organisation will derive immeasurable benefit from this section.

INTRODUCTION

When we are in a state of balance, we can realise our greatest potential in life. Optimal balance is a perfectly choreographed dance between arousal and regenerative states that allows us to grow and thrive.

Balance is becoming increasingly rare and perceivably impossible to achieve in today's world. Despite technology making our lives easier, we appear to have far less time. Professional and personal demands are relentless and all-consuming.

Admiration of success and intolerance of the mediocre are fast becoming the norm, and there is simply no allowance for failure. Expectation has replaced appreciation. Fairness and justice elude many, if not most. As the world gets smaller, family units are disintegrating, relationships have become disposable and social isolation continues to escalate despite advancements in social media.

It is little wonder that chronic stress has become highly prevalent in a world geared towards over-arousal. The stress response has always been vital to our very existence and survival. This highly energetic biological state enables us to adapt and even flourish in the most challenging of circumstances, but only under one condition – that it is activated sporadically.

Constant activation of the stress axis is not only systemically exhausting, it is damaging. It accelerates the ageing process, promotes pain and disease, and even compromises our ability to cope with change.

It is ironic that the very system that protected us for thousands of years, has now become one of the largest threats to our well-being and possibly even our future.

■

THE CENTRAL MESSAGES

This book does not promote stress avoidance or encourage disconnection from your daily life or society in any way. The narrative does not prompt you to change profession or even to adopt lifestyle habits that are impractical, let alone unrealistic. The reason for this approach is twofold.

The first lies within the definition of the word 'stress'. The Oxford English Dictionary offers the following: [noun] A state of mental or emotional strain or tension resulting from adverse or demanding circumstances; [verb] *Subject to pressure or tension.*

According to a study by researchers at the Yale University School of Medicine and at the University of California, the average individual living in developed society is likely to experience between four to five episodes of stress every week (1). We can never completely remove *adverse or demanding circumstances* from our lives. Essentially, life is one demanding and challenging circumstance after another. Likewise, we'll always be subjected to *pressure or tension.* The question is simply: how much and for how long?

Knowing this, we need to adjust our expectations of the world we live in and the society we're part of. We also need to adjust the expectations we have of ourselves.

The second reason that this book does not promote stress avoidance is because stress is potential. Many of our greatest accomplishments are born during times of challenge. Stress promotes personal growth and emotional development. Stress is often the driving force in our greatest triumphs in life, whether they be educational, physical or professional. Often stress forces us to break out of our comfort zones to create new and exciting realities. Stress also forces us to find creative solutions and can even change the course of our lives for the better, whether we realise it at the time or not.

Is it possible that our greatest achievements are not born in balance, but during acute stress?

STRESS AND POSITIVE LIFE CHANGES – A PERSONAL NARRATIVE

Looking back, I can fully identify and appreciate the profound influence that some periods of stress have had on my life. Although not pleasant at the time, and certainly not something I would consciously choose, many of these experiences pushed me in directions of growth and lifelong change. There is one specific event that will stand out forever.

IN THE MID-2000S, I was working for a highly ranked (top 10) tennis player, who was exceedingly popular due to his good looks, incredible talent and celebrity entourage.

Following the grass court season, I returned to South Africa for lecturing engagements at one of the local universities. During my absence, the player sustained a right shoulder injury. Not being able to return to the US immediately, I suggested he seek help from local therapists. We agreed to resume treatment on my return, which was a week before the start of the US Open. Confident that it was only a minor setback, I didn't think much of it and focused my attention on my students and local work commitments.

On the day of my return to the US, I contacted the player to find out how he was. To my surprise, he was still in pain, despite several weeks of treatment. I thought nothing of it because the first half of his year had been fairly smooth sailing and many of his physical challenges and injuries had been quickly and effectively managed. I reassured him that there was nothing to worry about, convinced that a week was more than enough time to manage the situation.

I arrived in New York on the Sunday morning. Instead of resting up and managing my jet lag,[1] I took the free day to meet up with friends and enjoy the city. The energy and excitement of New York got the better of me. Great restaurants, trendy bars, stylish clubs – I was having the time of my life.

The next day, the tennis star called to inform me of his arrival in New York, requesting that I meet him downtown where he was staying at a famous celebrity's apartment. I was feeling very groggy from my previous day's adventures. It was going to be challenging to focus on the impending briefing and treatment session. However, this did nothing to dampen my excitement. The apartment where the player was staying belonged to a famous blonde actress who was at the peak of her career – I couldn't wait to get there. (Of course, I was hoping that she would be there too.)

Once in the apartment, my attention was everywhere but on the task at hand. I was captivated. The photos on the walls, the furniture and the styling – it was all just incredible.

The player and I found a private room in the multi-storey apartment. He gave me a breakdown of recent events – the nature of the pain, the type of treatment he'd received and his frustrations. From his description, it seemed cut and dried – nothing I couldn't handle.

The athlete was eager to be assessed, diagnosed and successfully treated. There was one problem however – I couldn't find a single abnormality within the broader joint complex. At the time, it did seem strange, but I assumed that it was my lack of clarity as a result of jet lag and the previous night's adventures.

Still in my overconfident and carefree headspace, I decided to cover all bases and simply treat the entire region, no matter how big or small! This approach was the ultimate hedge, sure that one of the techniques would facilitate an improvement.

The session was nothing short of a marathon and probably the longest I have ever performed – yet to my surprise, there was neither an improvement in the player's range of motion nor his pain levels! It was then that my adrenalin[2] kicked in. My heart rate shot up. I began breathing faster and I could feel tension build throughout my entire body. Knowing professional athletes and their intolerance of failure, I became exceedingly anxious. The conversations in my head became all-consuming. Repeatedly, I attempted to reassure myself that this was not a crisis – yet. I still had some time.

We agreed to follow up the treatment session the next morning. This time I was fresh and focused – my job depended on it, as did my career! The second session was the same as the first. It was random, non-specific and I was still struggling to identify the origin of the mystery pain. During the session I sensed the player's frustration turning into irritation. As I was soon to find out, he was seriously considering finding my replacement.

After two marathon sessions there was still no progress. I didn't understand the pathology and could offer no explanations, let alone a prognosis. I was completely perplexed and, quite honestly, downright embarrassed. The US Open was in less than a week. This, compounded by the fact that the player had not been able to practise or train, made the likelihood of his competing very remote.

Before I left the apartment, he made it clear that he was going to explore various options in light of the lack of progress. I had no response and sheepishly left the apartment wondering where I went wrong. What was I missing?

By this stage, my adrenalin had been pumping non-stop for two days and cortisol[3] had saturated my system (known as the stress hormones, adrenalin and cortisol are covered in detail later in the book). I returned to my hotel in a complete state. It wasn't long before I received the call I was dreading. In light of the high stakes – endorsements, sponsors and rankings – the player had decided to bring in a new team from Europe that night. I was instructed to stay in New York until the weekend when we would meet again to re-evaluate our working relationship.

I was in complete overdrive mentally and physically. I couldn't sleep. I couldn't eat. It was impossible to relax for even a moment. Free time in one of the most exciting cities in the world held no appeal.

I could not stop thinking about his case. I must have run through the details of his shoulder pathology over a thousand times – it just didn't add up. Although working in high-level professional sport is an exciting and rewarding professional path, I must always bear in mind that my career is based on my last success, word of mouth and reputation – nothing else.

This scenario could signal the end of my career: being unable to resolve a seemingly remedial injury in a highly ranked 'celebrity' tennis player just before his most important competition of the year!

As my stress levels steadily climbed, my imagination got the better of me and I envisaged a mandatory change in career. Although I knew nothing about being a short-order cook, I thought a job in the burgeoning fast-food industry might be the next best career choice for me.

Despite the anxieties and fear, the stress response induced by this crisis did have a unique upside. I had more energy, as well as an increased oxygen and glucose supply to my brain. What I needed to do at this point was channel this elevated state into productive pursuits. It was then that I made a conscious decision to identify – or certainly try – the x-factor in the complex and currently unresolved shoulder pain syndrome.

I rushed out to the closest medical bookstore and searched high and low for an answer. The elevated adrenalin and cortisol in my system made my search seem effortless. A few hours into the search, I stumbled across a book entitled *Visceral Manipulation*[4] by a renowned French osteopath, Jean Pierre Barral. The book described unexpected relationships in the body, where compromised mobility of internal organs and their surrounding ligaments had the ability to induce joint and/or muscle pain through nerve circuits. It was fascinating. In my over-revved state I soaked up the information. The book described a very specific relationship between the liver – including its supportive ligaments and casing – and the right shoulder. More importantly, the book highlighted that a direct intervention could eliminate the pain, or at least reduce it. These anatomical relationships made perfect sense.

Excited by this discovery, I rushed back to the hotel and practised the various manipulations on a friend. My technique was poor, my understanding non-existent and my hands far from ready to tackle such a delicate and precise job on one of the best athletes in the world at the time. But this didn't faze me – I wanted another chance.

Five long days passed and finally the phone rang. I was summoned to the celebrity pad. Nervous at the outcome and reconciled to the potential reality of changing professions, I rushed downtown. The difference between this trip and the one six days earlier was that, instead of being lethargic and complacent, I was focused and motivated.

I was so focused on the impending meeting that I got out of the taxi on the wrong side of the road. While not a major issue in itself, I forgot to close the door and it was sheared off by a passing car! Despite the cab driver's outburst and the ensuing chaos, I just kept going. My adrenalin was working for me, my attention focused on one thing to the exclusion of all else.

I nearly tripped over the suitcases of the specialist European team at the entrance to the apartment. As they headed out, the mood appeared strained and the player seemed distressed.

Without hesitation, I was briefed on the week's events. The player's shoulder actually appeared less stable. Withdrawing from the tournament seemed inevitable.

Boldly I said, "Let's give it another go. We have nothing to lose." Reluctantly he agreed. Here was my opportunity. I threw everything at it. Every shoulder technique I have ever practised, heard about or seen was part of the treatment protocol. Not ideal, but this was a testing time. Finally, it was time for the visceral manipulation I had been practising all week. My technique was crude, clumsy and, in hindsight, way too aggressive. Nevertheless, my enthusiasm and focus overshadowed these shortcomings.

Once the marathon treatment was complete, we agreed to speak the following morning to decide whether withdrawal from the tournament was necessary. Needless to say, I didn't sleep at all. After the longest night of my life, the sun came up and my fate in professional sport was about to be decided.

Around mid-morning my phone rang. The player didn't greet me. There were no pleasantries, just an abrupt instruction to get across town. We were headed to the courts to practise. Yes, practise! The player had made a remarkable overnight recovery and was eager to get to the court as he was playing his first match the following day. Without going into too much detail, I repeated this treatment several times during the tournament. Incredibly, he reached the quarter-finals, mostly pain-free and playing exceptional tennis.

The following year, I enrolled in the world's foremost visceral osteopathy programme and committed to spending six to eight weeks a year with the pioneers in the field for the next decade. This additional and unique skill set increased my value as a health professional in the realm of professional sport, and propelled me to greater heights than I could ever have imagined.

The main protagonist in this life-changing event was stress. It gave me the ability to adapt to change, overcome challenging environments and find solutions in chaotic circumstances due to enhanced mental and physical acuity. Without this biological response, my professional growth and future successes would not have been possible.

Instead of fearing and shying away from stress, we need to acknowledge that stress provides opportunity. By harnessing the biological effects of stress, you can ultimately achieve your greatest potential in life, whether in personal growth or professional achievement.

THE DECIDING FACTOR

We all know of people who seem able to bounce back from repeated failure, endure relentless stress and keep going with tireless tenacity. These people seem to have a gene the rest of us don't have. While there is certainly a genetic component, there are other contributing factors such as emotional flexibility and mental adaptability. In short, it's resilience. And resilience can be learned.

Because we cannot avoid stress, nor would we want to considering the potential value that stress offers, our focus must move away from complete evasion towards resilience.

For those who are currently in the throes of stressful life experiences, committing to new behaviours and a series of lifestyle changes – no matter how valuable – is not easy. These shifts require significant time and considerable effort and discipline. This is not an issue when we are burden-free and healthy. It is very challenging during acute or chronic stress.

The experience of chronic stress is typically associated with exhaustion, irritability, lowered immune functioning and poor coping mechanisms – all compounded by complete and utter overload. To make changes or take on new routines appears daunting and nearly impossible. However, we must consider the severe consequences of not implementing change at some stage in our life, especially if stress is an ongoing feature.

As will become clear in the book, acute stress has little or no effect on our health and well-being and, remarkably, can even have health benefits. However, chronic stress is nothing short of disastrous in terms of health outcomes across all domains. The literature on chronic stress is extensive and offers valuable insights. We can capitalise on this science by using the numerous interventions that have proven effective in both protection and resilience.

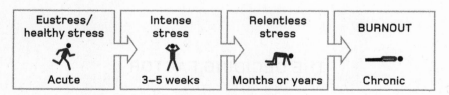

Figure 1 The stress continuum

2

THE SCIENCE OF STRESS

Scientists have been studying stress and its related health outcomes for over 70 years. Time and again, they've drawn the conclusion that we all intuitively know: Chronic stress has a negative impact on all aspects of health.

Researchers from the College of Physicians and Surgeons, and the Center for Behavioral Cardiovascular Health at Columbia University conducted an enormous systematic review and meta-analysis of the literature in the context of chronic stress and associations with the cardiovascular system (2). The review included six large observational studies involving 118 696 participants for over a decade. The review findings showed that chronic stress is associated with a 27% increased risk of coronary heart disease. This dramatically elevated risk is the equivalent of smoking more than five cigarettes a day or having high blood pressure and/or severely elevated cholesterol (LDL).

In an attempt to explain the association between chronic stress and the elevated risk of cardiovascular health issues, the authors suggest that disruptions in the hormonal and nervous systems, as well as weight gain, are largely responsible.

The negative health impacts of chronic stress are certainly not limited to the cardiovascular system. In fact, all major biological systems[1] are affected to some extent or another. This explains why chronic stress is typically accompanied by a diverse range of symptoms and ailments that often include muscle and body pain, colds and flu, behavioural changes and digestive issues.

In 2015, researchers at Harvard and Stanford universities published a collaborative meta-analysis involving 228 studies on stress and health implications (3). The study was able to determine a direct link between ten types of stress and four health responses, which included premature mortality and a decline in mental and physical health. The stress experiences included family conflict, work conflict, job insecurity, high job demands, lack of control in the workplace and poor social support.

What I found to be particularly interesting about this meta-analysis was the impact that conflict has on our health and overall well-being. The study showed that ongoing conflict is associated with a 90% chance of developing physical health issues. More concerning, it is associated with a 160% chance of developing mental health issues. While mental health issues are extremely difficult to manage in the medical space, another concern is the tremendous impact they are having on the world economy. The World Health Organization cites mental health issues as the leading burden on the world economy today. In fact, depression, which happens to be one of the more prevalent mental health issues, has been directly attributed to a loss of 74.9 million work days every single year – the single biggest impact on productivity in the world (4).

The Harvard and Stanford universities' collaborative meta-analysis also showed that job insecurity, high job demands and long working hours dramatically increase the risk of developing major health issues, which are associated with significant rises in premature mortality. Longer working hours, extended work weeks and less annual leave are more prevalent in the modern workplace, all of which, according to this study, appear to be having detrimental effects on our health.

In 2015, *The Lancet* journal published a study (5) on the relationship between long working hours and their impact on our health. The researchers analysed volumes of data from studies involving over 600 000 participants and found that, when compared with standard working hours of 35 to 40 hours a week, those who work over 55 hours increase their risk of having a stroke by 33%. There is also a 13% increased risk of developing heart disease.

In addition to alarming effects on all of our biological systems, by far the most disturbing impact of chronic stress is its impact on the integrity and stability of our genetic material, DNA. In short, **it damages our DNA**. Stress erodes and shortens the DNA telomeres – the protective protein complexes that cap our chromosomal[2] ends.

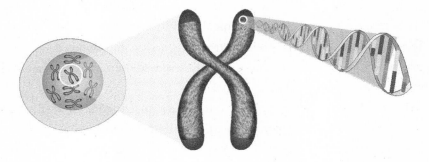

Figure 2 A chromosome with telomeres

Telomeres have several important functions. Firstly, they are responsible for organising our chromosomes in the centre of each cell. They are also responsible for preventing chromosomes from sticking together. But, most importantly, they protect our DNA during cell replication. When these genetic segments are prematurely shortened and eroded, numerous cellular issues result, including poor functioning, abnormalities, possible mutations, cell inactivity and even premature cell death. In fact, telomere erosion is believed to be one of the primary causes of both ageing and chronic diseases.

In 2004, Nobel Prize winner Dr Elizabeth Blackburn and a team of highly accomplished researchers published a study (6) on the impact of chronic stress on genetic integrity as measured by telomere length.[3] The study involved 58 women between the ages of 20 and 50. They were divided into two groups: those who had tangible, chronic stress in their home environments, and those who did not.

The study identified several important relationships between stress and genetic integrity. Firstly, those who had no appreciable stress in their home environments showed normal genetic structure, integrity and behaviours relative to their age. However, in the high-stress group, the destructive effect on telomeres and subsequently DNA was overt, but only under specific conditions. Those in the high-stress group who only experienced episodes of acute stress had little to no change in telomere integrity, whereas those exposed to chronic stress showed significantly compromised telomere length. Not only did the study's findings highlight the vast disparity between the effects of acute and chronic stress in terms of genetic compromise, accelerated ageing and trajectory towards disease, it also exposed the various mechanisms by which chronic stress induces this state.

The principal mechanism appears to relate to reduced activity and effectiveness of an enzyme called **telomerase**. This enzyme is exclusively responsible for maintaining the structural integrity and the rebuilding of telomeres, thereby promoting better genetic stability and enhanced cell division, functioning and performance. Whereas a telomere is a protein that maintains the stability of our DNA, telomerase is an enzyme that helps maintain the integrity of telomeres as well as rebuild their structure.

What this means for people who are exposed to familial stress over lengthy periods of time is that there is a strong association between chronic stress and accelerated ageing. In Blackburn's study, when the lowest-stress group was compared with the highest-stress group, the findings were dramatic. The highest-stress group had a degree of genetic compromise that correlated to an additional nine to seventeen years of biological ageing.

In other words, **stress shortens lifespan and increases the risk of developing age-related diseases**. It also accelerates our trajectory towards losses in functionality.

The discovery of **telomerase** is believed to be one of the most significant in recent medical history, especially within the areas of cancer and ageing. So profound in fact that Dr Elizabeth Blackburn and her two colleagues, Carol Greider and Jack Szostak were collectively awarded the Nobel Prize in Physiology or Medicine in 2009 (7) for their discovery.

Stress impacts our DNA not only as adults, but also as children. Over the last few years, several studies on adult participants have provided support for an association between a history of childhood stress, shorter telomere length and poor health outcomes during later stages of life.

Stress affects children and adults in much the same way. The difference lies in the increased impact some facets of chronic stress have on a developing child. Stress during early development affects aspects such as height, overall health profile, and mental and emotional integrity in later life. In effect, chronic stress has substantial, long-term implications.

In 2011, researchers from the Ohio State University College of Medicine published a study (8) showing that multiple childhood adversities were related to both elevated systemic inflammation and significantly shorter telomeres. Within the sample group of 132 healthy, older adults, it revealed that when compared to the absence of adversity, the level of genetic compromise could translate into a 7- to 15-year difference in lifespan!

The mechanisms underlying genetic compromise and accelerated ageing in response to stress are highly complex and multifactorial at any stage of life. Firstly, stress raises systemic inflammation, specifically in response to adrenalin spikes. Not only does chronic stress result in persistently elevated levels of inflammation, research shows (9) that individuals with early-life stress have a heightened inflammatory response to psychosocial[4] stress. Simply put, if your circumstances were challenging and stressful as a child, your inflammatory response in reaction to stress as an adult may be completely disproportionate.

Inflammation is part of the body's immune responses. It helps to protect us against harmful microorganisms, such as viruses and bacteria, as well as foreign bodies like chemicals and pollution. Inflammation is an integral part of the healing process after an injury or physical trauma. Without an inflammatory reaction, the body would not be able to heal damaged tissues.

Chronic inflammation occurs when the body activates an inflammatory response to a perceived internal threat that does not require this response. There is an increase in the activity of white blood cells. With no threat to deal with and nowhere to go, over time they can start attacking internal organs or other vital tissue and cells.

Persistent inflammation[5] has been linked to numerous health conditions including diabetes, heart disease, bone disorders, respiratory disorders, digestive compromise and mental health issues, such as depression.

Stress is also strongly associated with increased free radical[6] production. This elevated state of oxidative stress[7] can lead to increased telomere erosion and compromised genetic integrity. DNA, and telomeres in particular, are highly sensitive to damage by free radicals. However, in human studies it appears that this destructive relationship between stress and free radicals is bidirectional. Not only does stress increase free radical production, free radical exposure increases our susceptibility to stress, and can create disruptions in our biological responses to stress (6).

Cortisol has been shown to have a profoundly negative effect on genetic integrity. Cortisol contributes to telomere shortening by inhibiting the actions of the enzyme telomerase. In a 2008 study (10) researchers from the David Geffen School of Medicine at UCLA discovered that cultured cells exposed to cortisol showed significantly lower telomerase activity.

Supporting these findings, researchers from Stanford University, the University of British Columbia, the University of California and other prestigious medical institutions found that simulated stress in a group of five- and six-year-olds resulted in shorter telomeres, suggesting that early cortisol exposure may be a driver in premature biological ageing (11).

When combining the effects of elevated cortisol, increased free radical production and increased inflammation, it should come as no surprise that people appear to age rapidly in response to compounding life traumas.

THE INEVITABLE PHYSICAL BREAKDOWN

Without a doubt, long-term stress makes us feel unwell. Although stresses are constant throughout life, there are often specific times and situations where the degree and duration of stress exceeds our physical and emotional tolerance, with disastrous health consequences.

IN 2007, I WAS HIRED as the athletic director for the Chinese Olympic team in preparation for the Olympic Games to be held in Beijing the following year. I remember every detail like it was yesterday.

I landed at Beijing Capital International Airport towards the end of China's brutal winter, when temperatures can reach −20°C/−4°F! The airport had recently been rebuilt and gave the impression that Beijing was no different from any other major city in the world. After collecting my bags, I went to the arrivals hall expecting a friendly, helpful representative to meet me there and take me to the Olympic training centre, where I would be briefed and inducted into this exciting new chapter of my life.

As it turned out, there was no one there to meet me. I couldn't speak the language, no one spoke English, and all I had was the email address of the translator who facilitated the employment agreement. After hours of confusion, anxiety and stress, a driver approached me and finally I was on my way.

The drive was an adventure in itself. The car was definitely not roadworthy. The driver probably didn't have a licence and the traffic and impatience on the roads bordered on hysteria. After three chaotic hours, we finally arrived at the Olympic training site. It felt like a military barracks – armed police at the gates and throughout the centre. In broken English, the driver told me to keep my passport on me at all times and proceeded to show me to the dormitory where I would be staying.

The challenge at this point was breathing. The air was rough and metallic. The best analogy is that of trying to breathe in a basement parking lot in which all the cars are running simultaneously. I began to panic.

Once we reached my spartan quarters, the driver pointed towards a long corridor and gestured something that I took to mean 'food'. I managed to find the dining hall by following the trail of athletes. Once I got there I had no clue what to do and no one volunteered assistance. To top it all, I was the only foreigner in the centre so was subjected to some distrustful glares.

After dinner, I found my way back to my quarters to take a shower. The bathroom was a little different to what I expected – readers who have been to cheap hotels in China will know what I mean. There were no towels, no soap and no grip on the floor. Within minutes, I had taken a hard, bone-bruising tumble and had lacerated my shin on a broken tile. Bleeding, limping and battling to breathe – pollution still getting the better of me – I scrambled out of the bathroom to the bedroom, where I proceeded to patch myself up. Fortunately, I had a first aid kit with alcohol swabs, plasters and a broad-spectrum antibiotic. There was no one to call and certainly no doctor to consult.

The next day I was introduced to my superiors. They weren't charming and barely managed to be civil. Protocol was described abruptly. My responsibilities demanded a seven-day working week trailed by a film crew who would monitor my every move, and a weekly debriefing of my work every Sunday afternoon.

The culture of the team was to show no weakness. The policy was clearly zero tolerance! In a conversation with senior officials, I was told, "You push them hard all the time, and if they get injured or break down, we will replace them." I was soon to find out the same was true for me. I was certainly not going to mention the previous night's fall, would do my best to hide the limp and would change pants more regularly to hide the bloodstains that kept seeping through.

The team members were distrustful of foreigners so it took months to build even the slightest relationships. The administration proved ruthless and intolerant. To make matters even more challenging, outside communication and interaction was limited to email. I seldom left the training centre, had no local telephone number, the Internet was very poor and social media was banned.

The ongoing social isolation, having no sense of control, 70-hour working weeks and high job demands had my stress hormones in overdrive. My body eventually collapsed. I had flu more often than I shaved. I lived on painkillers, anti-inflammatories, antibiotics and antihistamines – my kidneys are still in recovery! But the hardest part was hiding all my ailments from the administration in the early stages of my employment.

THE STRESS RESPONSE – A SYSTEM IN CONFLICT

Despite the overwhelming research on the negative impact of stress on our health and, of course, society's negative perception of *big, bad stress*, there are many instances in which stress can enhance our functioning and performance, both physically and cognitively. The fundamental difference between the beneficial and the destructive effects of stress depends on a critical factor – **duration**.

Stress in short bursts (acute stress) protects, strengthens and enhances our abilities. It is important to understand that the stress response is one of the reasons we have been able to survive the most hostile of environments for thousands of years. The stress response is a strong biological reaction to danger or perceived threat, which is able to integrate all the major systems[8] of the body as a unified force to create powerful defences – instantaneously! In an instant, this protective response:

- releases enormous amounts of energy
- increases the availability of oxygen
- enhances muscle power
- promotes pain resistance
- provides mental acuity and strong immune defences.

Essentially, the true purpose of this highly organised biological force is to help us cope better with change and successfully react to emergencies. We are primed for success in this state.

Hyper-vigilance and metabolic overdrive provide the platform for accomplishment and successful adaptation under acute conditions, but as you know, chronic stress has detrimental health outcomes. Significant health compromise, together with a decreased life span, become more likely as constant engagement of this hyperactive biological state of stress exhausts the nervous, cardiovascular, hormonal and immune systems, leaving a trail of damage.

Societal changes over the last 40 years have transformed our once-essential protection system into the primary catalyst in health compromise!

UNDERSTANDING THE BIOLOGICAL PROCESS

The stress response happens in two distinct waves. The first is known as the sympathetic-adrenal-medullary (SAM) axis. The second is known as the hypothalamic-pituitary-adrenal (HPA) axis. Both have very important and unique roles, yet their biological effects are very different.

The first wave – SAM axis

The stress response begins in the amygdala[9] in the brain with the perception of a threatening or, more commonly, disturbing situation. The amygdala, which is involved in emotional processing, immediately sends a distress signal to the hypothalamus. Much like a command centre, the hypothalamus then rapidly mobilises the 'emergency' response through a branch of nerves that connects the brain to the adrenal glands. The adrenal glands respond to the call to action by pumping out adrenalin[10] to the extent that there is a 300–500% spike when compared with resting levels.

Adrenalin has a profound influence on our body as it is both a hormone and a neurochemical. It causes our heart rate, respiration and blood pressure to increase, improves circulation to the brain and limbs, releases energy into the bloodstream, promotes the release of endorphins[11] and mobilises our immune system into action. It also gives us super-senses, such as better smell and eyesight. All this happens instantaneously, faster than our visual processing centres can process change, which is why we can often react before the situation unfolds.

In ancestral times, periods of stress were typically accompanied by real physical threats. Part of the preparation for injury or impending infection would be increased potentiation of immune defences. Most stresses in early human history were life-threatening. The body compensates for this by changing the profile of the immune system in such a way that it is better equipped to protect against infection, secondary to body trauma.

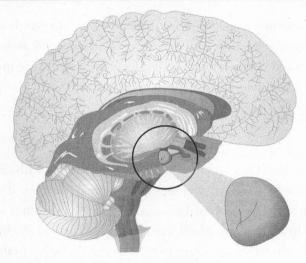

Figure 3 The amygdala (emotional response centre)

At this point you may be thinking: "How can this be bad? There is certainly no downside to having more energy, being mentally sharper, physically stronger, having strong immune defences and feeling no pain!" Well, it's not that simple. In order to prime the body for action and heightened responsiveness, several systems need to be shut down. You simply can't have it all.

One of the functions of adrenalin is to direct blood away from the skin, as well as the digestive and reproductive systems. Because reproduction and food consumption are unlikely to help in any significant way during acute stress, these systems are shut down in favour of enhanced performance by the brain, the cardiovascular system and the muscular system.

Have you ever noticed that when you are having a stressful time, you develop issues with your digestive system? Cramps, bloating and constipation are all symptoms of elevated adrenalin. A 2011 study by German researchers (12) showed that stress not only reduces blood supply to the gut by up to 400%, but also affects movement of the intestines and the secretion of enzymes, lowers regional defences and alters the composition of bacterial colonies that reside in the gut. Although other stress hormones may disrupt digestive and organ integrity, adrenalin appears to be the primary protagonist.

> Many people today suffer from long-standing digestive disorders and fertility issues, which are proving difficult to treat by conventional means. The research shows that *chronic stress is a major contributing factor* in the onset and duration of these types of health disorders.

Elevated adrenalin also impairs the body's regenerative, reparative and growth potential. As an adult with low physical demands, one can get away with this, at least for short periods of time. However, the big concern is our children. Chronic stress is becoming increasingly more prevalent in adolescents. Higher demands, greater expectations, technology, information overload and lower activity levels all contribute to impaired growth, a weaker physical profile and a greater predisposition to pain syndromes and health ailments. This may be most apparent in their late teens, as they approach adulthood.

In adults, a big concern with repeated adrenalin surges is the impact they have on the cardiovascular system. According to renowned neuroscientist and world authority on stress, Dr Bruce McEwen, adrenalin surges result in a dramatic rise in blood pressure, which can damage blood vessels in the brain and heart. The arterial damage creates rough zones where plaque can accumulate, resulting in restricted blood flow and arterial hardening. It is no coincidence that chronic stress has such strong associations with increased risk of heart attack or stroke.

The second wave – HPA axis

Following the initial adrenalin surge, centres in the brain produce hormones that signal the adrenal glands to produce a second hormone, cortisol.

In the short term, cortisol has a very positive effect on our immune system. Adrenalin mobilises the immune system into action, cortisol improves responsiveness and helps to regulate function. Without cortisol to balance adrenalin's mobilising effect, the immune system could become overactive and potentially destructive.

As with everything in life, balance is important. While cortisol regulates immune behaviour in the short term, in the long term we see a very different picture. Long-term elevations of cortisol lead to immune system suppression, predisposing us to latent viruses and infections, which is why we often get sick after long periods of stress.

There is even more complexity within this biological process. Recent discoveries by Sheldon Cohen and his team from Carnegie Mellon University (13) show that chronic elevations in cortisol create a resistance of cells and tissues to the actions of cortisol. This can manifest in several inflammatory-mediated diseases, and potentially even life-threatening autoimmune[12] disorders.

Essentially, the prolonged presence of cortisol can either suppress our immune system or completely fail to regulate it, both of which are extremely antagonistic to health.

Not only does cortisol impact immune functionality, it also has a diverse influence on our body. This includes:

- increased activity levels
- disrupted sleep patterns, especially when cortisol is elevated late in the day
- demineralisation of our bones
- muscle breakdown
- excessive gastric acid secretion, resulting in heartburn and reflux, and
- altered brain chemistry.

Cortisol's effect on body composition

From an energy balance perspective, high cortisol levels increase fat storage. In fact, cortisol can lead to significant weight gain, despite good dietary habits. It does this through various channels, which include:

- increased appetite
- reduced sensitivity of the body's cells to insulin[13]
- reduced levels of growth hormone.[14]

It has been well established in the literature that chronic stress can lead to changes in eating behaviours that can include changes in food preferences and timing of meals, as well as an increase in overall consumption (14).

According to Finnish researchers, the negative mood states that typically accompany stress, such as depression, anxiety, irritability and fatigue are highly correlated with an increase in food intake (15). Something we have all experienced at some point in our lives.

Not only does a stress-induced shift in affective mood trigger a robust appetite, but at the same time, it triggers a reduced desire to be physically active.

If the radical changes in appetite and tendency towards reduced physical activity weren't enough of a challenge to the waistline, consider that according to studies in the *Journal of the Academy of Nutrition and Dietetics* (16) and *The American Journal of Clinical Nutrition* (15) chronic stress also tends to elicit cravings for sweet and fried foods, soft drinks and alcoholic beverages.

With all these compounding factors, it is little wonder that chronic stress is often associated with either weight gain or shifts in body composition.

In the same way that many people gain weight during times of severe and persistent stress, others lose weight. The reason for this inconsistency may lie in the prevailing dominance of either the SAM or the HPA axis, and the corresponding elevations of stress hormones.

When cortisol dominates, weight gain is likely; however, when the sympathetic nervous system and adrenalin dominate, weight loss is common. The reasons for weight loss include ongoing release of energy into the body from existing reserves, reduced gastric motility[15] and appetite, as well as increased activity levels. Interestingly, according to a study published in *The International Journal of Obesity* (17), when men are confronted with high job demands, low control and ongoing strain, those with a low Body Mass Index (BMI)[16] have a tendency to lose weight (SAM), whereas those with high BMIs gain weight (HPA).

Cortisol's effect on the brain

One of the greatest concerns with chronic stress is cortisol's effect on the brain. In 2012, researchers from the departments of Psychiatry and Neurology at Yale University published a study (18) showing that chronic elevations of cortisol are associated with lower mass in regions[17] of the brain responsible for executive function, complex intellectual behaviour, self-awareness, coordination and even motivation.

Interestingly, this was not the first study to show the negative effects of cortisol on brain tissue. Extensive research on animals and humans shows that the memory and emotional centres[18] are particularly prone to compromise in terms of structure and functioning.

The brain is divided into two primary cell types – grey matter and support cells known as glia, and white matter. Grey matter is densely packed with nerve cell bodies and is responsible for the brain's higher functions, such as thinking, computing and decision-making.

White matter consists of axons, which create a network of fibres that interconnect neurons and create a communication platform between brain regions. White matter gets its name from the white, fatty myelin sheath that surrounds the axons, and speeds the flow of electrical signals between neurons and brain regions.

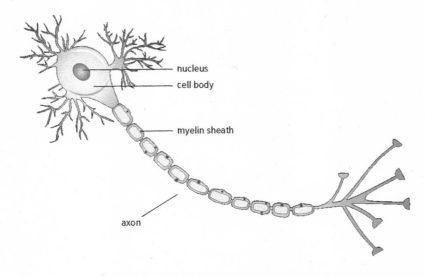

nucleus
cell body

myelin sheath

axon

Figure 4 The structure of a human nerve cell (neuron)

Although the literature shows that elevated cortisol causes brain cell shrinkage and premature death, neuroscientists at the University of California have discovered another way in which chronically raised cortisol influences the brain. Daniela Kaufer and her team discovered that cortisol could also trigger stem cell[19] malfunction, changing the overall composition of the brain (19).

According to Kaufer and her team, chronic stress and corresponding spikes in cortisol can cause overproduction of white matter and reduced grey matter. This creates a major compositional disruption that spills over into function.

The study focused on a specific region of the brain known as the hippocampus[20] that is known to atrophy during periods of chronic stress.

In adults, stem cells in the hippocampus typically mature into grey matter. However, this study showed that under conditions of chronic stress, when cortisol is raised for protracted periods of time, these stem cells mature into white matter. This change in brain composition can cause significant functionality issues later or even in the long term, which may explain why chronic stress is associated with reduced learning ability, compromised memory and a dramatic decline in cognitive potential.

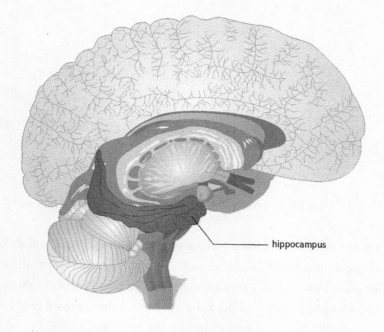

Figure 5 The hippocampus

Kaufer also discovered that the increase in white matter increases the connectivity between the two primary emotional centres – the hippocampus and the amygdala. A hyper-connected emotional circuit perpetuates a vicious cycle by creating more rapid and extreme fear responses. This predisposes us to a more constant state of fight-or-flight, resulting in more cortisol production and even greater neurological pathology (brain compromise).

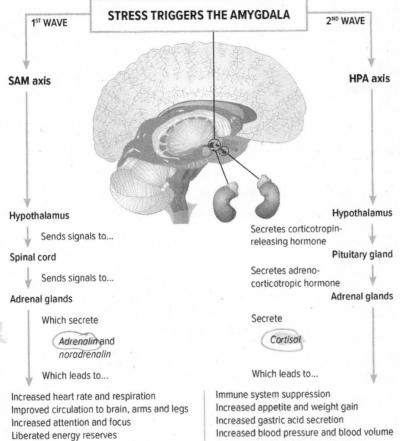

STRESS TRIGGERS THE AMYGDALA

1ST WAVE

2ND WAVE

SAM axis

HPA axis

Hypothalamus

Sends signals to...

Spinal cord

Sends signals to...

Adrenal glands

Which secrete

Adrenalin and
noradrenalin

Which leads to...

Increased heart rate and respiration
Improved circulation to brain, arms and legs
Increased attention and focus
Liberated energy reserves
Faster metabolism
The release of endorphins
Mobilisation of the immune system
Increased blood pressure
Reduced blood supply to the skin,
reproductive, digestive and auditory
systems
Reduced kidney function

Hypothalamus

Secretes corticotropin-
releasing hormone

Pituitary gland

Secretes adreno-
corticotropic hormone

Adrenal glands

Secrete

Cortisol

Which leads to...

Immune system suppression
Increased appetite and weight gain
Increased gastric acid secretion
Increased blood pressure and blood volume
Reduced motility of the intestines
Breakdown of muscle/tendons and
demineralisation of bones
Reduced bone formation, muscle growth
and repair
Lowered serotonin, brain-derived
neurotrophic factor, thyroid hormone
and growth hormone
Brain shrinkage, alterations in brain
composition, disrupted connectivity
Psychological and emotional issues
Compromised learning ability, poor memory,
focus and attention

Figure 6 Stress and the amygdala

Although the emotional centres become increasingly well connected, the same is not true elsewhere in the brain. Kaufer found lower than normal connectivity between the emotional centres (especially the hippocampus) and the prefrontal cortex, a region of the brain that moderates our perception of stress.

With lowered connectivity to the rational brain, and hyper-connectivity of the emotional centres, it is no wonder that our behavioural patterns during periods of chronic stress become nothing short of hyper-emotional, illogical and even atypical.

The collective effect of brain cell shrinkage, premature brain cell death, altered connectivity and reorganisation of brain tissue is dramatic within the behavioural and cognitive space. This will typically manifest in:

- poor focus
- impaired memory
- short attention span
- loss of goal orientation
- antisocial behaviour
- anxiety
- fear, and
- general emotional instability.

I am describing an average person on an average day!

CHAPTER SUMMARY

- The effects of acute (short lived) and chronic (protracted) stress are vastly different.
  - Acute stress protects, strengthens and enhances our abilities. It helps us cope with change and respond successfully to emergencies.
  - Extensive research confirms that chronic stress exhausts the body and has a profoundly negative effect on all aspects of health.
  - Work stresses, such as long working hours, high job demands, conflict, lack of control, insecurity, and poor social support negatively influence life expectancy, physical health, general well-being and, most notably, mental health.
  - Mental health issues have become the leading burden on the world economy, partly due to lost productivity and partly due to the increased burden on healthcare systems.
- Chronic stress damages our genetic material (DNA), speeding up the ageing process and increasing the prevalence of many chronic diseases.
- Chronic stress can induce biological changes that equate to 9 to 17 years of additional ageing.
- Children who experience chronic stress may experience long-term genetic compromise that may translate to a 7- to 15-year shorter life expectancy, if not addressed later in life.
- Early life stress creates hyper-reactivity of the stress axis, creating a greater propensity towards systemic inflammation.
- Simplified, the stress response is divided into two waves or component parts:
  - The **first wave** is the instantaneous fight-or-flight reaction initiated by the hypothalamus. This reaction is referred to as the

sympathetic-adrenal-medullary (SAM) axis.

- It is associated with a strong and rapid activation of the sympathetic nervous system and the release of adrenalin. Increased blood pressure, heart rate, respiration and immune activity typically accompany this initial response.
- Prolonged activation of the first wave has detrimental effects on the digestive, urogenital, immune and cardiovascular systems.

▫ The **second wave** is referred to as the hypothalamic-pituitary-adrenal (HPA) axis and is associated with the release of the hormone cortisol.

- While sporadic cortisol release improves immune functionality, long-term elevations create immunosuppression and, in some extreme cases, a complete failure to regulate immune behaviours; this may lead to inflammatory and autoimmune diseases.

■ Chronically raised cortisol:

▫ leads to a breakdown in numerous bodily systems, and digestive issues

▫ results in weight gain, abnormal eating behaviours and reduced insulin sensitivity

▫ causes the brain to shrink, disrupts the composition of the brain, creates disconnection between various parts of the brain, and results in damage to the very regions that manage the entire stress response

▫ impacts our memory, focus, attention, cognitive potential and even levels of motivation.

STRESS IN THE WORKPLACE

■

THE WHITEHALL STUDIES

According to the American Institute of Stress,[1] the work environment is the primary source of stress for those of us living in developed countries.

Perhaps this is why the medical community's attention has been increasingly drawn towards the social determinants of health. Two acclaimed studies performed by Sir Michael Marmot, a Professor of Epidemiology and Public Health at University College London, have provided extraordinary insights into stress and health outcomes.

The Whitehall studies monitored approximately 28 000 British civil servants over a 40-year period. The studies confirmed for the first time that stress in the workplace directly affects health and lifespan – again, something we intuitively know.

More importantly, the Whitehall studies (20) identified that the grade of employment[2] was one of the most reliable predictors of perceived stress and increased risk of mortality from a wide range of diseases.

Logically, we would assume that senior, high-ranking employees would be more prone to health issues, due partly to increased responsibilities and partly to seniority in age. However, the study showed the exact opposite. It was the lower-ranking employees within the organisation who had the worst health and highest risk of premature death. In fact, those in the lowest-ranking positions had a 300% higher risk of mortality when compared to the most senior employees over the ten-year period of the study.

Several years later, the second of the Whitehall studies (Whitehall II) (21) confirmed these findings. However, this second study was able to identify why this was the case – in essence, it cracked the stress code. The researchers showed that the lower-ranking employees had less social support, less variety at work and, most importantly, an overwhelming sense of lack of control when compared with those in more senior positions. What the study identified was that the highest perceived levels of stress, and consequently the greatest degree of health compromise, were in environments where control is lacking.

Supporting this assertion, in a 2015 meta-analysis (3), Harvard Professor Jim Goh and Stanford Professor Jeffrey Pfeffer describe a lack of job control to be the leading cause of premature mortality (>40% greater risk) within the broader framework of stress. So much so that it overshadows the stress-health implications of unemployment (40% increased risk) and work or family conflict (20% increased risk).

Triggers in stress

Recent research has turned conventional wisdom within the context of stress and health outcomes on its head. The notion that a high degree of life pressure and responsibility promotes stress and is associated with poor health outcomes has been notably proven incorrect. This is just as well, seeing that responsibilities and pressures in life appear to be on the rise, and there are no indications that this will change any time soon. According to a 2014 report by the American Psychological Association and the American Institute of Stress (21a), 48% of people living in the US say their stress has increased in the last five years. There is no reason to believe that this data doesn't apply to other industrialised nations as well.

While chronically high demands can be independently associated with compromised health, it is the combination of high demands and a lack of control that appears to be one of the greatest drivers in stress and its wide range of negative health associations.

If we reflect on our experiences of stress throughout the course of our lives, a sense of lack of control has accompanied almost every challenging situation. However, the Whitehall and several more recent studies have identified many other major factors in the promotion of this biologically exhausting state, whether in a professional environment or in our personal lives. Some of the more profound factors in the workplace include:

- a lack of fairness, or injustice
- a lack of, or poor, social support
- social isolation
- an effort-reward imbalance, and
- a lack of authority over day-to-day decisions.

Either independently or in combination, each factor contributes to over-activation of the stress axis and progressively erodes our core health.

Although the Whitehall and many of the offshoot studies focus on the corporate environment, Sir Michael Marmot believes that they provide far more than merely an insight into professional behaviours and health outcomes. Rather, they serve as a template for society at large.

The impact we have on those around us is far greater than we realise, and if we wish to reduce societal stress and negative health associations, we need to start with ourselves. Improving our behaviour and treatment of others can dramatically impact their well-being in both the short and long term.

Marmot believes that 40 years of research, involving tens of thousands of people, has shown that societal stress and its negative health associations can be significantly reduced by:

- allowing people to feel that they have more control in their lives
- encouraging and supporting skills development and education
- always rewarding positive behaviours
- allowing others to be involved and participate in communal decisions
- always promoting fairness and a sense of justice in both the workplace and at home, and
- always championing and encouraging fair treatment of others.

So often we are fixated on our own agendas and lives that we don't realise the profound influence we have on others. This powerful message highlights the larger responsibility we all have to improve the lives of those around us, with the ultimate beneficiary being society.

Leaders create the culture

High-stress professions are no longer the exception, they are the norm. Enormous losses in intellectual capital are ravaging organisations every year. According to the "World Health Organization methods and data sources for global burden of disease estimates 2001–2011"(4), mental health issues are the leading disease burden and account for the single greatest cost to economies in both developed and developing nations. Consider that data captured in 2014 by the American Psychological Association and the American Institute of Stress shows that 73% of people experience psychological issues due to stress.

The 2017 report on work-related stress by The Health and Safety Executive in the United Kingdom showed that in 2016 12.5 million working days were lost due to stress, depression and anxiety. The same statistics review points out that 40% of all ill health cases and 49% of all working days lost due to ill health can be attributed directly to stress.[3]

Without question, stress contributes to disengagement at work, higher absenteeism rates, reduced productivity and greater staff turnover.

With the intention of improving corporate health profiles and increasing productivity, the second Whitehall study and other more recent studies outlined a model that emphasises more employee involvement in decisions, improved social support in the workplace and ongoing reward for positive behaviours.

Promote a feeling of control amongst employees

According to the Harvard and Stanford[4] meta-analysis, lack of control in the work environment is associated with an elevated risk of reporting the following:

Poor physical health	>40%
Poor mental health	>40%
Physician-diagnosed health conditions	>20%
Premature death	>44%

A collaborative research report published a few years ago on the topic of 'premature exit from the labour market' showed that greater job control was a key component in employee retention (22).

A lack of control in the workplace has significant ramifications within the context of mental health. A 2008 Danish review of 16 studies involving no fewer than 63 000 participants found that low decision latitude strongly correlated with depressive symptoms or major depressive episodes, especially in men (23). When you consider that depression is a recurrent mental disease characterised by episodes of reduced mood and interest that persist for at least 14 days, the implications in the context of productivity losses and corporate burden are very clear.

Based on the evidence, the following policy guidelines are advised:

- realisation that improved working conditions could lead to

a healthier workforce, better employee retention and greater
productivity
- appropriate involvement in decision-making is likely to benefit
employees at all levels of the corporate structure
- reorganising practices to enable employees to have greater control,
and
- introducing mechanisms for measuring and monitoring employees'
level of control over their work.

Promote social support and justice in the workplace
According to the research (3), both lack of social support and unfairness have
significant negative effects on employee health and lifespan. The health statistics for lack of social support are:

Poor physical health	>35%
Poor mental health	>38%
Physician-diagnosed health conditions	>20%

Additionally, a lack of support from supervisors and unclear or inconsist-
ent behaviour are associated with a twofold increased risk of poor mental
health when compared with those in more supportive environments (24).
Interestingly, lack of social support has a greater influence on women than on
men in the workplace.

The statistics for unfairness/low organisational justice are considerably higher
in the mental health and physician-diagnosed health conditions categories:

Poor physical health	>35%
Poor mental health	>60%
Physician-diagnosed health conditions	>50%

In 2007, researchers from the Department of Epidemiology and Public Health at University College London and the Finnish Institute of Occupational Health published a study on unfairness and health (25). The study included data collected from twenty civil service departments in London and involved more than 8 000 participants over an eleven-year period. They came to the following conclusion:

> *Unfairness is an independent predictor of increased coronary events and impaired health functioning. Further research is needed to disentangle the effects of unfairness from other psychosocial constructs and to investigate the societal, relational and biological mechanisms that may underlie its associations with health and heart disease.*

Perceptions of unfairness have been found to be associated with dramatically increased levels of psychological distress. In a longitudinal study (26), researchers found that low justice in the workplace was associated with a 41% higher risk of absenteeism due to illness in men and a 12% higher risk in women.

The defined policy implications suggest that:

- improved levels of support from managers may reduce ill health and sickness absence
- work environments that facilitate mutual support between colleagues and do not tolerate antisocial behaviour promote health and well-being
- clear and consistent information from managers/supervisors can have a positive effect on employee well-being and health, and
- policies that promote fairness in the workplace are likely to result in improvements in health.

Create an effort-reward balance

Crucial to all social relationships is a sense of reciprocity. One-sided relationships have been shown to be a significant source of stress and associated illness.

Effort may come from your intrinsic drive or may be a prerequisite of your work environment. It is important to realise that the literature supports the belief that high effort by itself is neither stressful nor detrimental to health. As our grandparents used to say, hard work never killed anyone.

Reward within the professional domain is perceived and measured in not just one but three different ways. We typically assume that if we pay well, that in itself creates an effort-reward balance, but nothing could be further from reality. The literature shows that the three aspects that are critical to this balance are appreciation, career opportunities – including job security and promotion prospects – and, of course, financial compensation. Should any of these be lacking, the scale will be tipped, increasing stress and ill health in the workplace.

Confirming this assertion, an extensive review of 45 studies by Dutch researchers (27) showed that elevated stress and corresponding health compromise occur in those environments where effort levels are high and reward levels are low. The negative relationship between effort and reward is often referred to as an effort-reward imbalance (ERI).

The Whitehall II study found that an abnormal ratio of high effort in relation to low reward corresponded to a 36% increased risk of developing coronary heart disease and a 28% increased risk of suffering from a non-fatal heart attack. The impact of low reward on health was not limited to the cardiovascular system. Within the group of over 10 000 participants, a clear lack of reward dramatically increased the odds of developing poor physical and mental health! What's worse is that those with low social support at work or in the lowest employment grades showed the greatest degree of susceptibility to these health risks (28).

These findings have been replicated in several other European countries including France (*GAZEL-Cohort Study*), Sweden (*WOLF-Norrland Study*) and Germany (*Public Transport Employees Study*) (29).

Not only does a lack of reward impact company infrastructure from a health perspective, it also results in high staff turnover. In professions such as law, medicine and accounting, this can have devastating consequences on overall performance. A 2015 research report (22) showed clear evidence that lack of reward in the workplace influenced employee retention. According to the study:

We found that higher ERI was associated with exit from the labour market independent of age, sex, education, occupational class, depression and allostatic load.

Allostatic load is the wear and tear on the body that accumulates over time when an individual is exposed to repeated or chronic stress. It represents the physiological consequences of chronic exposure to the associated fluctuating or heightened nervous system and hormonal responses.

The same report found that reward in response to effort offered protection from premature exit from the labour market.

Based on the current body of evidence, the defined policy implications encourage:

- establishing a good balance between the effort expended by employees and their reward structure
- increasing praise, encouraging individual development and, where possible, raising salaries, and
- improving social support networks among colleagues.

More about clinical depression and anxiety disorders

As of February 2017, the United Nations Health Agency reported depression to be the leading cause of disability worldwide. According to an extensive report by the World Health Organization, the total number of people living with depression in 2015 exceeded 322 million, constituting 4.4% of the world's population (30). The trend in depression rates is even more disturbing. The report points out that the total estimated number of people living with depression increased by 18.4% between 2005 and 2015. Whether this reflects the overall growth in the global population or perhaps a growing ageing population in which depression is more prevalent, is difficult to say. Nevertheless, these figures are no less alarming.

Moreover, as mentioned earlier, the diagnosis of depression is not simply based on a slight alteration in mood for a day or two. There are several definitions of this psychological state, but typically it is characterised as a recurrent disorder that is associated with reduced mood and interest that persists for at least 14 days.

According to the World Health Organization:

> *Depressive disorders are characterized by sadness, loss of interest or pleasure, feelings of guilt or low self-worth, disturbed sleep or appetite, feelings of tiredness, and poor concentration. Depression can be long-lasting or recurrent, substantially impairing an individual's ability to function at work or school or cope with daily life.*

The proportion of the world's population suffering from anxiety disorders is also alarming. Anxiety disorders refer to a group of mental disorders characterised by feelings of anxiety and fear, including generalised anxiety disorder, panic disorder, phobias, social anxiety disorder, obsessive-compulsive disorder and post-traumatic stress disorder. Symptoms range in severity, but anxiety disorders are generally more chronic than episodic in nature.

The WHO reports (30) that in 2015 the total estimated number of people living with anxiety disorders was 264 million, accounting for 3.6% of the total population. As with depression, there has been a sharp rise in reported cases since 2005.

The Lancet journal recently published an article on the global, regional, and national incidence, prevalence, and years lived with disability for 310 diseases and injuries from 1990 to 2015 (31).

The article showed that, over a ten-year period, the incidence of anxiety disorders rose by nearly 15%. Statistically, females on the American continent have the highest global incidence, reporting as much as a 7.7% prevalence rate.

■

CHAPTER SUMMARY

■ Stress is on the rise – 48% of those living in the US report a rise in stress levels in the last five years.

■ Research shows that our work environment is the primary source of stress in our lives.

■ The breakthrough in the understanding of stress, specifically in the professional domain, came through two British studies, known as the Whitehall studies.

■ The Whitehall studies evaluated over 28 000 people over a period of 40 years, and identified a lack of control or a feeling of having no authority over decisions as the primary driver of stress.

■ A lack of control is associated with a greater than 40% risk of dying prematurely along with other significant health issues.

- Other key factors that contribute to stress are a lack of fairness, injustice, inadequate social support, social isolation, and an effort-reward imbalance.
- Studies reliably show that responsibility and high demands are not the cause of stress.
- We can change the world around us by making a conscious effort to lower our 'stress footprint'. To do this we need to:
  - give more control to those around us
  - support skills development
  - reward positive behaviours
  - allow for participation in decisions
  - always be fair
  - champion justice, and
  - provide support as and when needed.
- As many as 73% of Americans experience psychological issues due to stress.
- In the UK, 12.5 million working days are lost each year due to stress, depression or anxiety.
- Of all working days lost in the UK, 49% are attributed to stress.
- Mental health issues are the leading global disease burden and stress is considered a contributing factor.
- Team leaders, managers and executives should implement the following strategies to reduce illness rates, increase employee engagement and improve productivity:
  - Promote a feeling of control amongst employees through appropriate involvement in decision-making; reorganise practices to enable employees to have greater perceived authority.
  - Promote social support and justice in the workplace, discourage antisocial behaviour, facilitate mutual encouragement, always provide clear and consistent instructions, and advocate fairness.
  - Promote an environment where efforts and rewards are balanced.

Increasing rewards is more effective than reducing demands. This is achieved through the encouragement of individual development, increased praise and appreciation and, if possible, greater financial compensation.

▢ A change in corporate policies favouring stress reduction will reduce the global burden of mental health issues.

4

CRACKING THE STRESS CODE

ATHLETES AND STRESS

For almost two decades, I have worked in a professional environment that is saturated with stress. While the public sees only the glamorous aspects of competitive sport – large salaries, celebrity lifestyles and adoring fans – there is a very different picture behind the scenes.

Very few talented, aspiring athletes actually make it to the professional circuits. The career disappointments are relentless, and the final realisation that this is the end of the road within competitive sport is nothing short of brutal.

For those who do get to the top in their chosen sport, it has come at a huge cost: team politics where injustice is common, political agendas that take away control, and high public expectations routinely create stresses and anxiety for the elite athlete. And if that isn't enough, exhausting travel schedules result in long periods of solitude and fragmented relationships. And then there's the injury factor. Injuries destabilise earnings, impact endorsements, derail the athlete's position in the team and can even terminate an already short career.

It would be one thing if all of these pressures and tensions presented at a mature age when the athlete could intellectualise the daily stresses, but they don't. Great athletes start young – very young – and so does the stress and relentless strain.

Ongoing pain, constant fatigue, loneliness, isolation, disappointment, failures, financial pressure and uncertainty carve out the path to professional sporting success.

Yet this group is exceptionally healthy and seemingly immune to the adverse effects of chronic stress.

In 2014, Spanish researchers performed an extensive meta-analysis (32) of ten studies that involved data from a total of 42 807 athletes. The research team found that competitive athletes have a lower risk of cancer and cardiovascular disease when compared to the general population. They were also found to live considerably longer.

A few years ago, the *British Journal of Sports Medicine* published a study (33) performed over a 50-year period on 2 363 athletes and 1 657 controls. The aim of the study was to assess life expectancy, comparing various sports disciplines[1] to non-athletes. The findings showed that overall, high-level athletes live five to six years longer than non-athletes.

Fortunately, you don't have to train intensely for several hours a day, six or seven days a week to achieve stress resilience and longevity.

A recent study revealed that the exceptional health profiles seen in athletic populations might not be directly attributed to intense training. According to this 2012 analysis (34), athletes who participate in high- and medium-intensity sports[2] have the exact same health profiles and survival advantages as those who participate in low-intensity[3] sports. However, the study, which involved 9 889 Olympic athletes from 43 disciplines, did point out that the health advantages seen across the various sports disciplines did not exist in activities that involved repeated bodily collision and intense physical contact. In fact, that detracts from health, giving an 11% shorter lifespan.

How do athletes buffer extreme stress?

I have been involved with countless athletes at all levels within a variety of sports over the years. Living and working with these unique individuals has taught me many valuable lessons. I have learned about the value of intensity and an unyielding commitment to the attainment of goals and aspirations. I have seen average athletes become 'greats' through hard work, an ongoing desire to improve and a relentless will to succeed. However, the greatest lesson for me has been the way that they overcome the chronic stress that accompanies this life path.

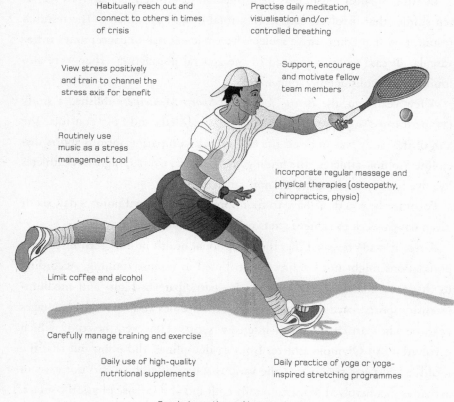

Habitually reach out and connect to others in times of crisis

Practise daily meditation, visualisation and/or controlled breathing

View stress positively and train to channel the stress axis for benefit

Support, encourage and motivate fellow team members

Routinely use music as a stress management tool

Incorporate regular massage and physical therapies (osteopathy, chiropractics, physio)

Limit coffee and alcohol

Carefully manage training and exercise

Daily use of high-quality nutritional supplements

Daily practice of yoga or yoga-inspired stretching programmes

Regularly use the pool to promote recovery and incorporate ice baths or contrast showers (alternating hot/cold)

Figure 7 Stress resilience habits of successful athletes

From a young age, these athletes are conditioned to see stress as a positive experience – an experience that not only promotes growth, but also brings out their greatest attributes and abilities.

Elite athletes cope with their stress by reaching out and connecting to those around them – all the time. Sport psychologists, coaches, physical therapists, trainers and even family members form a cohesive and collective unit that is constantly available to deconstruct events, offer advice, listen and provide support.

Guided relaxation, mental imagery, meditative techniques and breathing exercises are regular daily practices. Yoga-inspired stretching protocols may be performed several times a day, in and out of competition. Music, massage, physical therapies and even cold water immersion[4] are part of an ongoing routine.

Moreover, supplementary exercise activities and sports training are always carefully manipulated to promote the greatest positive hormonal[5] changes.

At the core of their routine is diet. Careful food choices that promote recovery, reduce inflammation, and provide energy and an abundance of nutrients are considered essential. Added to this is the prolific use of high-quality nutritional supplements. These nutraceuticals are carefully selected by medical experts and their intake perfectly timed to promote the greatest possible benefit.

Food additives, preservatives and other artificial ingredients are avoided where possible, as is alcohol. Caffeine is consumed only in moderation and at predetermined times – early in the morning or 30–60 minutes before training.

Intriguingly, many of these core practices remain after the athletes retire. It is little wonder that athletes are resilient to chronic stress and have enhanced longevity and lower disease rates. Could we, as part of a population suffering from the adverse effects of chronic stress, benefit from their behaviours and practices? Do they have an answer to the chronic stress epidemic that is costing the US economy over $300 billion annually? The science says YES! It affirms each and every aspect of their routines, individually and collectively.

A model for stress resilience

Two factors underpin the model for stress resilience that I present in this book: Working with and observing athletes and their seeming ability to withstand extreme ongoing stress, and a deep need to find out whether science confirms and supports what I instinctively know.

Stress resilience can be learned in four fundamental steps:

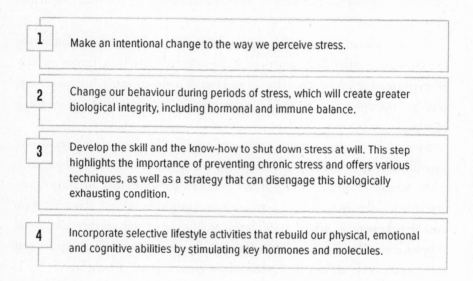

1   Make an intentional change to the way we perceive stress.

2   Change our behaviour during periods of stress, which will create greater biological integrity, including hormonal and immune balance.

3   Develop the skill and the know-how to shut down stress at will. This step highlights the importance of preventing chronic stress and offers various techniques, as well as a strategy that can disengage this biologically exhausting condition.

4   Incorporate selective lifestyle activities that rebuild our physical, emotional and cognitive abilities by stimulating key hormones and molecules.

Stress is a prerequisite in terms of growth, improvement and personal advancement throughout life. I have always held by the saying, "Nothing of consequence in life comes easily". Whether a challenging degree, aspirational job, meaningful relationship or even excelling in sport, advancement takes enormous effort and has many hurdles along the way. It is the hurdles in life that ultimately propel us to the next level. We cannot do this without the tools to harness the energies of acute stress and manage the destructive effects of chronic stress.

CHAPTER SUMMARY

- From a young age athletes are confronted with significant stress and seemingly relentless challenges. More often than not, ongoing pain, constant fatigue, loneliness, social isolation, disappointment, failure, financial pressure and uncertainty carve out the path to professional sporting success.

- Despite the ongoing stress and unremitting pressures that exist within their playing and competitive environment, for the most part athletes are exceptionally healthy and appear to be immune to many stress-related ailments and chronic diseases.

- A meta-analysis of ten studies that involved data from 42 807 athletes showed that sportspersons have a significantly lower risk of heart disease and cancer when compared to non-athletes.

- Research over a 50-year period shows that, on average, athletes live five to six years longer than non-athletes.

- Contrary to previous scientific beliefs, the stress-buffering capabilities and health advantages seen in athletic populations cannot be solely attributed to vigorous exercise/activity. Research shows that athletes competing in less-vigorous sports (such as golf and cricket) have the same health advantages as those engaged in more physically demanding activities (such as tennis and triathlon).

- The remarkable resilience to chronic stress and ongoing life challenges seen in athletic populations may be ascribed to a broader holistic approach that includes:
  - Viewing stress positively and training to channel the stress axis for benefit
  - Habitually reaching out and connecting to others in times of crisis
  - Routinely supporting, encouraging and motivating fellow team members

- The practise of daily meditation, visualisation and/or controlled breathing
- Incorporating regular massage and/or physical therapies (osteopathy, chiropractics, physio) into their weekly routine
- The daily practice of yoga and/or yoga-inspired stretching programmes
- The regular use of water-based modalities to promote recovery and fitness, which include swimming, ice baths and/or contrast showers (alternating periods of hot/cold)
- The consistent intake of high-quality nutritional supplements
- Structured management of sports training and supplementary exercise
- The limited consumption of coffee, alcohol and pharmaceuticals (unless absolutely necessary)
- Routinely following a healthy diet
- The regular use of music as a stress and performance management tool.

5

STEP 1: CHANGE YOUR PERCEPTION OF STRESS

Albert Einstein said, "Reality is merely an illusion, albeit a very persistent one." When it comes to stress resilience, perception is everything.

■

A NEGATIVE PERCEPTION OF STRESS IS BAD FOR YOUR HEALTH

One of the best examples of this is a study (35) that followed 28 753 adults over eight years to determine whether the belief that stress is bad impacted their health.

Part of the study involved a questionnaire that asked participants how much stress they had experienced over the previous year, and how much they believed that stress affected their health.

In terms of premature mortality and poor health outcomes, neither the amount of stress nor the perception that stress is bad independently predicted either to a meaningful degree over the eight-year period. However, the study showed that when a stressful event was combined with the perception that stress is bad for your health, it increased the risk of premature mortality by 43%!

The same study also reported that 33.7% of adults believe that stress affects their health to some extent or another.

To appreciate the health significance of this impactful study's findings, the research team from the University of Wisconsin used cumulative risk models to estimate the number of deaths attributable to this combination of stress and a negative perception of stress.

Based on these models, each year in the United States 20 231 deaths would be attributable to being stressed and believing that stress negatively affects health.

According to the 2013 Centers for Disease Control and Prevention (CDC) rankings, this would mean that the perception that stress negatively affects health is the fifteenth largest contributor to mortality in the US.

This is by no means the only study evaluating the relationship between the perception of stress and health, but it does show the profound impact of a negative viewpoint. The issue we all face is that wherever we look we are bombarded by the narrative of big, bad stress – and not without just cause. But this is not a balanced view, as stress can be a positive and necessary factor in so many of our experiences. This understanding has sparked a new wave of research into the reappraisal of stress as a necessary and protective biological experience. The irony is that the stress response has always been protective – we just haven't had the skills and know-how to adjust our response to it in modern times.

REFRAMING STRESS AS A POSITIVE EXPERIENCE PROMOTES HEALTH AND PERFORMANCE

In 2012 a team of researchers from Harvard University (36) examined how reappraising stress might influence cardiovascular functioning and attention/focus during and after a stressful simulation. The study involved 50 participants who were instructed that they were going to complete a public-speaking task.

Before the assignment the participants were divided into three groups:

1. Group I was assigned to an arousal-reappraisal model that consisted of instructions educating them on the functions of stress responses and encouraging them to interpret stress arousal as a tool that aids performance. Basically, the premise was that stress is good for you – don't fear it or see it as a negative biological response during challenges.
2. Group 2 received a placebo intervention that described the best way to cope with stress was to ignore the source of that stress. Simply put, the best way to rise to a challenge is to pretend or ignore the fact that you are stressed and that your system is aroused.
3. Group 3 was given no instructions.

During the stress simulation, only Group I showed significant changes in their cardiovascular system. This group had lower constriction of their blood vessels, thus lower blood pressure, and they also exhibited greater cardiac output.[1] Seeing that high blood pressure is associated with heart attacks and strokes, and that under non-reappraisal stress conditions blood pressure does increase substantially, the health implications are incredible. These effects on the cardiovascular system both protect our health and enhance our ability to function. The study also found that attention and focus were greater in Group I, the reappraisal group.

Not only can viewing stress as a positive experience protect our health and enhance our attention, research by Harvard's Jeremy Jamieson (37) has shown that stress reappraisal facilitates improved biological recovery from stressful episodes. In other words, it improves the body's ability to recover from challenging events and situations. This is especially significant in that the major trigger in health compromise associated with chronic stress is a progressive inability to shut the stress axis[2] down.

These two studies show that a simple shift in perception can protect the areas of the body that are most susceptible to stress-induced compromise. Adjusted perception can also enhance our ability to perform in and under pressure. That said, my favourite study is yet another Harvard publication, only this time the focus was on academic performance under pressurised conditions. Whether we are athletes competing, scholars writing a test or professionals writing board exams, the ramifications of these findings are life-changing.

The study, entitled "Turning the knots in your stomach into bows: reappraising arousal improves performance on the GRE"[3] (38), showed that a simple shift in stress perception could improve academic test scores. The study recruited 60 students preparing to take the rigorous exam. Half of the participants were informed that the signs of physiological arousal, such as increased heart rate, increased respiration and muscular tension that accompany testing situations predict better, not worse, performance. The other half of the group was essentially a control group and were given no information or instructions. The research team set up a practice exam for the entire group. Before beginning the practice test, all the participants provided a saliva sample that was analysed for alpha amylase, a protein enzyme that can collectively determine levels of dopamine, adrenalin and noradrenalin. These are key neurochemicals that promote and facilitate attention, focus and cognition.

Remarkably, the group assigned to reappraise stress arousal showed an increase in alpha amylase, and improvements in their performance on the quantitative section of the practice test, relative to the control group.

But that wasn't the main narrative of the study. What was absolutely incredible was the fact that one to three months following the practice session, participants returned to the laboratory with their score reports from the actual exam. Compared with controls, on average, the reappraisal participants scored higher on the test and reported that arousal on the day of the test had aided their performance.

While ongoing research in the area of reappraisal of stress is showing consistent findings of health promotion, protection and performance enhancement, the mechanisms driving its translation into physiological responses are not well understood.

The primary lesson from this literature is the *power of the mind*. We can't always control the stressors that confront us every day, but we can certainly control the way in which we perceive them. This gives us considerable authority over our health and performance.

A **stressor** is an external stimulus or an event that causes us to feel stress that results in a rise in adrenalin and cortisol. This may happen in a variety of situations that include environmental (pollution, loud sounds, heat), dietary, pharmaceutical, social and physical challenges, as well as interpersonal dynamics.

Within the context of the human body, a **trigger** is something that either sets off a disease in people who are genetically predisposed to developing the ailment, or that causes a certain symptom to occur in a person who has an existing disorder.

Perception – a personal journey

CHANGING MY OWN PERCEPTION of challenging events has not only allowed me to manage my personal stress better – it has also positively influenced my life. I can recount so many meaningful situations, but the most memorable was as a naval recruit in the winter of 1991.

Throughout my schooling, I worked as a waiter most evenings, the principal motivation being financial independence. This led to a very unhealthy lifestyle. My days were filled with school and whatever I managed to take in, and my evenings with work. Proper nutrition, vigorous exercise and sleep were sacrificed, but I had youth on my side and took full advantage. By the time I had finished high school towards the end of 1990, I had managed to save enough money for a five-month holiday in the US, before my military service[4] was set to commence.

Several relatives who had emigrated to the US in the late seventies kindly offered accommodation and an opportunity to experience the American way of life.

My expectations were certainly not aligned to reality, but in my defence, a teenager's expectations are seldom met. Immersed in suburban America, without a car and unable to experience the cool bars and clubs I had seen on TV – partly due to a drinking age of 21 and partly because I had no friends – it wasn't long before I became unfulfilled and self-destructive.

My days were spent sleeping until midday, eating copious amounts of junk food, especially thick-based, over-cheesed pizza, consuming kilograms of sugar and watching hours of mindless TV. I thought I was having the time of my life, yet in hindsight the adventure that I had planned turned out to be nothing like I imagined. While these lifestyle practices can certainly do no harm for a week or two, the picture that unfolded four months later was nothing short of disastrous.

I had gained weight, become lazy, lacked all motivation and the thought of work, exercise or studying was completely removed from my mind, which had probably shrunk by that stage. My social skills had also suffered. I became agitated, irritable and, frankly, depressed. Yet, for whatever reason, I still believed I was having the time of my life and living the dream.

Thankfully, it was soon time to return to South Africa, although the thought of military service was terrifying. I knew that the physical demands would be tough, so I decided to give myself a week to get into shape before the impending intake. Back in South Africa, I hit the road for a full ten minutes on at least three occasions – after all, I didn't want to be overtrained! Like any super athlete would, I fuelled my sessions with sugars, refined carbohydrates and loads of processed cheese – not wanting to lose the skills I had gained abroad.

Intake day arrived. The journey began with a bus ride – a long one – eighteen hours of suspense and excitement heading into the unknown. It was at this point that my stress levels began to elevate. The first trigger was the level of fitness and slick military-style haircuts apparent in the bus. Did I miss the brief? I have never felt more out of control or underprepared in my life. My heart did not stop pounding the entire eighteen-hour ride.

We finally arrived at the Saldanha Naval Base. The setting was magnificent – huge sand dunes and turquoise ocean. I thought to myself that this would make a great resort and, for a moment, was excited to be there. As we all got off the bus, the bomb hit – as did the screaming! At first, the screams weren't ours – they came from a group of young drill instructors – but after an hour of shuttle runs they were ours.

With my lack of fitness, it felt like my lungs had literally exploded! My legs couldn't propel me, which had nothing to do with the wind resistance caused by my long, wild hair. Too stressed to eat on the journey, I wasn't among the recruits who repeatedly ejected their stomach contents. What seemed strange at the time was the 10-second rule. This unreasonable and less-than-practical instruction was given to any distance the group had to run: 80 metres – we had 10 seconds; 100 metres – we had

10 seconds. I am not sure if the leading seaman – the 17-year-old charged with our care – knew that the world record was only a fraction faster. We didn't have spikes, starting blocks or low-resistance shorts. Instead, we ran in normal shoes, long pants that chafed and a collared shirt. Needless to say, we never met targets and just kept running.

Finally, after a briefing at 11 pm on the various rules and protocols that were in effect on the base, the day came to an end. Just as well I was used to little sleep from my schooling days, because four hours later the dorm of 30 men was woken up to loud noises – banging of aluminium pots and firecrackers! Was this a surprise party for us? If it was, it was a running party that included a few steel beds, a sand dune and 30 tired men.

Two hours later, it was time for our dorm inspection. The inspections routinely involved shaving skills, dorm hygiene, bed-ironing skills and uniform integrity and cleanliness. Needless to say, there was beach sand all over the floor, our beds weren't made, our uniforms were immersed in sand and sweat, and most of us had the odd bristle or two on our faces. Out we went again, only this time it was for an early morning winter swim in the cold Atlantic Ocean. The leading seaman was kind enough to allow us to keep our kits on while doing push-ups in the ocean, which were followed by sprints in our wet, salty uniforms.

Finally, by 7 am the ordeal ended, and we were all sent to the showers to clean up. The outside temperature was a nippy 10°C/50°F and we were all freezing. Looking forward to a hot shower, we entered the bathrooms walking like cowboys – in less than 24 hours an angry rash had already entrenched itself on our inner thighs – only to find the leading seaman waiting. In the few hours I had known him, I realised that nothing good ever came from this character, who was fortunately dismissed several weeks later due to abusive conduct. Huddled together, shivering and exhausted, we were informed that there would be no hot water for the duration of the winter. Cold shaves and cold showers followed for the next three months.

My initial naval experience was made worse by the fact that I was always at the back of the group during training or drills due to my extreme lack of fitness. This, combined with my poor discipline, did not make the environment any easier for me.

It wasn't long before basic training got the better of me. I felt socially isolated, there was no justice in this world, and nothing was fair. I felt completely out of control. Three of the four major stress drivers were a constant.

The days and nights were overwhelming. My body ached everywhere; I was exhausted, run down, depressed and anxious. I felt sorry for myself, and I constantly complained about the hardships, but no one had the desire or capacity to listen.

An additional knock occurred about three weeks into basic training. Our group, which consisted of several hundred servicemen, was gathered on the parade ground for an address by the base captain, a man not known for his way with words or charisma.

The captain announced that a certain percentage of deaths during basic training was considered acceptable and reminded us that no national serviceman would be leaving basic training prematurely without dying, being court martialled or dishonourably discharged due to mental health issues.

The address amplified my current psychological state, characterised by extreme self-pity. The strain and decline in my vitality steadily continued, although I did manage to develop a few skills, like anonymity.

One Saturday afternoon there was a big rugby match on, which both officers and non-commissioned officers wanted to watch.

This gave us some much-needed downtime. The base was serene. Having the rare opportunity to walk and not run, I went for a stroll to clear my head, and to take in the magnificent setting. That moment was the turning point, not just in my naval experience, but for the rest of my life.

Realising that I had two more years of national service, I made a conscious decision to change my mindset. No longer was I going to feel self-pity and indulge this negative emotional state brought on by my current circumstances. I decided then and there that I was going to always be positive, embrace the daily challenges and try my best regardless.

Incredibly, the transition was almost instantaneous. Within a week I was in front of the group in all drills and training exercises. I began to thoroughly enjoy the experience and even thrive! As training became increasingly more rigorous and demanding, I became mentally and physically stronger. My relationships with my fellow recruits drastically improved and for the next two years I literally had the time of my life – so much so that I signed up for an additional year of service. I do not recall being injured, sick, depressed or even run down after that defining moment.

Had I not changed my mindset that day, I would not have incorporated many important disciplines into my life. The positive shift in perception revealed an intrinsic ability to thrive under pressure and the true power of inner strength.

I have come to acknowledge that were it not for that one moment, my life would have been very different. A simple change in perception was the catalyst for this incredible metamorphosis. Interestingly, I never went back to my old ways. I am up by 5 am, usually earlier, exercise daily, watch what I eat – most of the time, at least – and have had the same haircut since 1991.

CHAPTER SUMMARY

- There are two facts that we cannot ignore: Stress is unavoidable, and perception is reality. So how we perceive stress becomes the reality we respond to.
- Stress resilience requires that we re-evaluate and adjust our perceptions of stress.
- It is difficult to change our perception of big, bad stress because it is supported and reinforced everywhere in our society. However, science now sees acute stress as positive in that it is a necessary and protective biological experience.
- Research has shown that when a stressful event is combined with the perception that stress is bad for your health, it increases the risk of premature mortality by 43%!
- Not only can viewing stress as a positive experience protect our cardiovascular health and enhance our cognitive abilities, stress reappraisal improves our body's ability to recover from challenging events and situations.

6

STEP 2:
CHANGE YOUR BEHAVIOUR

We've discussed how the stress response is associated with an increased release of adrenalin and cortisol into the bloodstream. According to research published in numerous medical journals, stress within a variety of different contexts also triggers the release of a hormone called oxytocin.

Oxytocin has powerful effects on both our psychological and physical well-being. It is now understood that oxytocin release during stressful situations serves to dampen physiological stress levels. In other words, it creates biological balance during a state of crisis. Yet, until recently, very little was known about this hormone other than its association with childbirth, human bonding and maternal behaviour. If you think about it, from a physical and emotional standpoint, childbirth is the single most stressful point in a woman's life, which happens to be the time when oxytocin levels spike the most.

An article entitled *"The role of oxytocin in social bonding, stress regulation and mental health: an update on the moderating effects of context and inter-individual differences"* (39) points out that when oxytocin is administered to healthy subjects, subjective stress ratings decline and stress hyper-reactivity diminishes. This is partly due to the fact that oxytocin has both direct and indirect inhibitory effects on the amygdala (40).

However, oxytocin's effects on our biology don't stop there. In 2005, Swedish researchers published a paper (41) on the effects of oxytocin in the context of healing and protection. Their paper highlighted the powerful influence that oxytocin has on behaviour and perception-of-self. The hormone promotes self-worth, confidence, fearlessness, optimism, a sense of calm, generosity, connectedness, and empathy towards others – an ideal profile for success in any endeavour, let alone stress buffering.

Intriguingly, this is the opposite psychological profile to the one induced by elevated levels of cortisol. Prolonged periods of raised cortisol promote fear, anxiety, emotional instability, antisocial behaviour, and so on. Essentially, **oxytocin acts as an emotional antidote to stress**.

From a physical standpoint, oxytocin's effects are even more profound. Oxytocin is linked to lowered cortisol, lowered heart rate and lowered blood pressure, thereby counteracting the common effects of the stress response. Additionally, oxytocin has anti-inflammatory actions, antioxidant effects and increases the production of serotonin and nerve growth factor (NGF). These are all key elements in healthy brain functioning. According to the study, oxytocin also increases levels of insulin growth factor 1 (IGF-1), an important hormone that promotes growth and repair of the body. Collectively, these effects provide a platform for vastly improved physical and cognitive integrity.

THE BIG QUESTION

If oxytocin has so many positive effects on our behaviour and physical integrity, why is it that we are not completely immune to the negative effects on our health attributed to chronic stress? The answer lies in the biological half-life of oxytocin. Scientists have discovered that oxytocin is rapidly metabolised in the human body and loses half its initial effectiveness within 1–6 minutes.

If we are to derive benefit from oxytocin for its stress-buffering effects, we would require more frequent surges. This would require the hypothalamus' and the pituitary gland[2] to be stimulated regularly. To add complexity to this biological scenario, oxytocin is principally released only in the initial stages of the stress response.

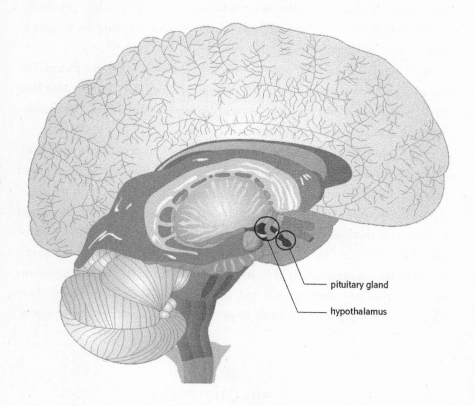

pituitary gland

hypothalamus

Figure 8 The hippocampus and the pituitary gland

Social psychologist Dr Shelley Taylor from the University of California (42), together with other medical researchers, was able to shed light on the role of oxytocin release in stressful situations. Taylor speculates that the release of oxytocin in response to stressful stimuli is to direct our behaviour to seek support from others, connect to others and feel empathy for others in times of crisis. There are two major benefits of this connection. The first is that we handle stress and life's challenges better as a collective, and the second is that when we connect with others either physically or socially, we trigger the release of more oxytocin, which promotes considerable physical and psychological resilience to stress.

Oxytocin is unlike any other hormone or neurochemical in the body in that it is a pro-social hormone. This means that the bonds with others determine the magnitude and frequency of release.

The physical triggers in oxytocin release include physical contact with others such as hugging, light touch, massage, and eye contact. Another mechanism by which we increase oxytocin levels is through pro-social behaviour. Caring for others, giving to others and feeling empathy towards others, all trigger oxytocin release.

Caring for others

In 2013, Michael Poulin at the University of Buffalo and a team of researchers from other institutions published a study entitled *"Giving to others and the association between stress and mortality"* (43). The study monitored 846 participants over a five-year period. Participants completed baseline interviews that assessed past-year stressful events and whether they had provided tangible assistance to friends and/or family members during this time. Mortality rates were assessed through access to public records.

The study revealed that for every major stressful life event, there was a 30% increase in the likelihood of premature death. However, the study also showed that participants who provided care for those close to them had no negative health outcomes following major life stressors. In simple terms, attending to the needs of others promotes incredible stress resilience, and the mechanism that has been identified in facilitating this protection is oxytocin release. Several subsequent studies support these findings.

Charity

Giving tangible care or assistance to others is not the only pro-social trigger in oxytocin release. In 2013, the journal *Hormones and Behavior* published a longitudinal study focusing on the function of oxytocin as a biological mechanism for buffering the adverse effects of chronic stress (44). The two-year study gathered data from 1 195 participants between the ages of 18 and 89. The participants were evaluated for their degree of charitable behaviour, which included donating blood, donating money to or volunteering for a charity, attending a community group meeting and so on. The total number of these activities was used to evaluate the overall level of charitable behaviour. Over the following two years, the participants provided information pertaining to stressful life events as well as physician-diagnosed physical ailments.

Remarkably, the results of the study clearly showed that greater charitable behaviours buffered the associations between stressful events and the onset of health ailments among the participants – largely through oxytocin pathways. Simply put, the more you give to others the greater the health protection you have during stressful periods in your life.

The study also revealed several important discoveries related to oxytocin and genetics. The research showed that individuals with diminished oxytocin sensitivity due to specific genetic variants[3] are more prone to stress-related physical health problems. So much so that stressful life events reliably predicted the onset of health ailments in this group. By contrast, those without these genetic variants[4] had absolutely no association between stress and ill health, which further emphasises the powerful influence that oxytocin has in the context of stress buffering. Incredibly, when it came to charity, those who had the genetic predisposition to abnormal oxytocin sensitivity, and therefore the highest health-risk profile in response to stress, benefited the most.

Now we know why some people handle stress better than others. Those who have genetic issues with oxytocin uptake in the brain don't cope well with stress and become ill. The study points out that even if you have a genetic variant that compromises your ability to handle stress, charitable behaviours can increase uptake.

Pro-social behaviour is not only associated with a rise in oxytocin levels, but also activation of the parasympathetic[5] nervous system. The mechanism by which this systemic balance is achieved is principally by activation of the vagus[6] nerve, one of the most important regulators of body processes.

Compassion and verbal support for others

In 2015, researchers from the Universities of Toronto, Arizona and California conducted four separate studies involving 300 participants on the effects of compassion on the human body (45). All four studies showed that the experience of compassion when encountering the suffering of others leads to lower cortisol levels, lower heart rate, lower blood pressure and reduced inflammatory markers. The beneficiary of the compassion is likely to experience similar effects. These biological changes occur largely through activation of the parasympathetic system, by means of increased vagus nerve activity.

Not only can compassion buffer the adverse effects of stress, it appears that expressing support and affection can have the same biological outcome. A study published in the journal *Behavioral Medicine* (46) investigated the effects of supportive communication and the verbal expression of care during and after periods of stress. During stress simulations, researchers found that those who expressed care and provided verbal support to loved ones had significantly reduced cortisol levels and heart rate responses. In fact, the degree of expressed support and care was a reliable predictor of cortisol output under these stress simulations.

The team of researchers from Arizona State University found that stress hormone levels return to baseline far quicker following the expression of care for others than under normal conditions. Participants in this study (47) were exposed to a series of simulated stressors and were subsequently assigned either to an experimental group or to one of two control groups. Those in the experimental group were asked to write a letter to someone close to them in which they expressed their feelings of affection for the person. Those in the first control group were instructed to think about a loved one without engaging in any communicative behaviour. The second control group sat quietly. All three conditions were compared according to stress hormone levels, namely cortisol. The results showed that, compared with the control groups, the participants in the experimental group experienced accelerated cortisol stabilisation/recovery following exposure to the stress simulations. Simply put, expressing care for others facilitates a speedier recovery from stressful events.

EARLY IN MY PROFESSIONAL SPORTS CAREER, I had the privilege of working with the captain of the national rugby team, the Springboks. He was iconic then and still is today. He was certainly not the largest guy on the field, but he played with the biggest heart and led by example. People always asked me, "What makes him so good?" and "How did he compete against guys so much bigger than him week in and week out?" The answer lies in our discussion on charity and compassion.

As a great captain, he constantly encouraged his teammates, and showed them support and compassion both on and off the field. What's interesting is that, by doing so, he was lowering his inflammation levels, lowering his stress hormones and improving cardiovascular functionality, which also supported his recovery from matches and training.

■

THE IMPACT OF ALL THE PRO-SOCIAL BEHAVIOURS ROLLED INTO ONE

Emily Ansell of the Yale University School of Medicine and Elizabeth Raposa of the University of California recently published an insightful study on pro-social behaviour and its relationship to stress and health outcomes (1). The study involved daily assessments in the evening, prior to bedtime. To ensure compliance and accurate data, research assistants monitored survey completion. Each evening, participants were asked whether they had experienced any stressful life events during the course of the day, and if so, were asked to record the number of events they experienced. Stressful events were drawn from a wide variety of domains that included work, health, finances and family events. The total number of stressors experienced across all domains was used as a measure of the daily stress burden.

At the same time, participants were presented with an established list of pro-social behaviours[7] and asked to disclose all the helpful behaviours they engaged in during that day. The measure of pro-social behaviour was the total number of positive behaviours engaged in each day.

The positive and negative affects[8] of the day's events were measured using the 10-item short-form of the Positive and Negative Affect Scale[9] (PNAS). During the evaluation, participants rated the extent to which they were experiencing different positive and negative emotional states. Based on their ratings, the positive and negative affect subscales were calculated. Daily mental health was also measured through a rating scale ranging from 0 (poor) to 100 (excellent).

Taken as a weekly average, the participants experienced approximately four to five major stress events and engaged in about eleven pro-social behaviours. As would be expected, those who experienced greater-than-average stress reported more negative emotional states and worse-than-average mental health.

Without taking stressful events into account, higher-than-average daily pro-social behaviour was associated with positive outlooks and better overall mental health.

More importantly, when looking at the relationship between stress and pro-social behaviour, researchers found that pro-social behaviour moderated the relationship between daily stress and overall mental health. In the study group, those who reported the lowest levels of pro-social behaviour also reported the greatest susceptibility to stress, negative emotional states and reduced mental health.

Change your behaviour – change your life

FOR THE BETTER PART OF the year, I had been based at the Olympic training centre in the heart of Beijing. Preparations for the Olympic Games were intense and the air was highly charged – China had to win at home. I have to admit that, as a foreigner, the team were wary of me - I didn't speak the language, I was unfamiliar with the culture and I made no attempt to engage beyond the requirements of my work portfolio. The days were not easy. My circumstances were challenging due to social isolation, demanding hours, a total lack of control over my schedule, elements of inconsistency in administrative decisions and even animosity on the part of the team who worked under me – they all wanted my job!

Working in the South African sports environment had conditioned me to approach my work with a rigid and uncompromising style. *My way or the highway* – after all, I was accountable for the outcome and I did my utmost to control as many variables as possible.

By this point in the year, many of the injured athletes had

recovered and their performances had started improving. All indications were such that my role within the team would be more valued and I would be given greater decision latitude and a little bit of breathing room, so to speak. This was not the case. A clash of styles and clash of wills were ever present, as was the threat of the discord escalating.

As the days passed, I found myself becoming more introverted, more disconnected from my working environment and longing for my old life on the professional tennis circuit. That life had been very different from my spartan existence in Beijing. Almost every week the entire tennis tour community moves to a new and exciting city. We are driven around, stay in the best hotels and eat at great restaurants. By taking the job in China, I had traded those comforts for a room containing little more than a wooden desk, a single bed and a small cupboard. Trendy restaurants had been traded for a super-sized mess hall with hundreds of athletes!

In June of 2008, I was sent to Wimbledon to accompany the Chinese Olympic tennis team. They were an incredible group of young ladies who were about to experience major career breakthroughs. Being back at Wimbledon was invigorating. I had returned to the professional world I knew and loved. However, being in London amplified my negative feelings about my current role and circumstances in Beijing. I wanted to be back on the tennis tour. At least I thought so at the time. It was great to see friends and fellow South Africans, to be able to speak the same language, to go out in the evenings, have access to social media and, without a doubt, I loved working in professional tennis.

As the tournament was drawing to a close, I started feeling down and dejected. The thought of returning to Beijing and facing those hostile conditions on a daily basis was more than distressing. One evening, I was sitting on a stationary bike in the gym – I'm not sure if I was actually cycling or just sitting when I noticed one of the most iconic figures in tennis and women's rights get onto the bike next to me. Incidentally, a movie has recently been made about her life – it was brilliant.

I knew the player fairly well because she is a personal friend and mentor of a former Number 1 player I had worked for. After an initial greeting followed by a few minutes of silence, she leaned over to me and asked what was wrong. Here was my gap, someone who would listen to my poor-me story. Without hesitation or restraint, I began complaining about my current professional circumstances and personal challenges. Expecting a receptive audience and a sympathetic ear, her response was very surprising.

I was expecting acknowledgement of my predicament with a smidgen of compassion. That wasn't the case. Instead, she said, "Listen to me carefully. There are two things you must realise in life if you want to be a success. The first is that pressure is a privilege and the second is that champions adapt." She went on to explain that no one in a position of great responsibility, or who is under significant professional pressure, is there because they are average. We must embrace these opportunities, not shy away from them. She also explained that all winners in life adapt. They change according to the circumstances they are in rather than resist them. In this way, they are able to grow and move forward.

Although it was not what I wanted to hear at that exact moment, I respected her as highly accomplished and one of the all-time greats.

For a day or so I processed what she had said and decided that I was going to make some personal changes on my return to Beijing. I took her advice to heart. By then, I fully realised and appreciated the importance of my position. Irrespective of the challenges, to be in a leadership role with one of the greatest sports teams in history was more than an honour, greater than a privilege, it was a once-in-a-lifetime opportunity.

Up until that point, adaptability had been sorely lacking in my repertoire of life skills. I decided I was going to make a concerted effort to change my behaviour. This meant becoming more flexible at work and more flexible in relationships. I tried to learn Mandarin as best I could and I completely immersed myself in Chinese culture.

I can say with absolute conviction that from that point on, my personal and professional experience in China was transformed. The next two and a half years were some of the best years of my life – I loved every moment. As my relationships with the administration and the athletes grew, trust began to blossom. With that trust, I was given greater latitude to make decisions, which equated to more control in my life and considerably less stress.

It has been established that social support during life stresses offers substantial coping and health benefits. However, it had been assumed that receiving support is the primary driver in this symbiotic relationship between people. What the latest research reliably shows is that engaging in pro-social behaviour as well as the bonds that form as a result, may be the most effective way of buffering stress that we know of.

Ongoing engagement in pro-social behaviour influences numerous health-promoting biological processes, including the oxytocin system (48), the reward circuitry in the brain (49), and most importantly, it activates the vagus nerve, which shuts down the stress response and promotes the restoration of balance and functioning in all major organs and hormonal systems (50).

CHAPTER SUMMARY

- Science has shown that by elevating oxytocin, we can counteract many of the damaging effects of chronic stress.
- Oxytocin has direct and indirect inhibitory effects on the amygdala, the fear and emotional response centre in our brain.
- Oxytocin also has a powerful effect on behaviour and perception of self. Oxytocin promotes:
  - self-worth
  - confidence
  - fearlessness
  - optimism
  - a sense of calm
  - generosity
  - connectedness
  - empathy towards others.
- Oxytocin also protects our nervous system, brain and circulatory system because it:
  - lowers cortisol levels, heart rate and blood pressure
  - has anti-inflammatory actions and antioxidant effects
  - increases nerve growth factor.
- Oxytocin increases insulin growth factor 1, which promotes growth and repair in the body.
- How do we increase our levels of oxytocin? It is triggered by physical contact and pro-social behaviours such as:
  - massage and body therapies
  - hugging
  - handshakes
  - prolonged eye contact
  - intimate relations.

- Actions we should specifically introduce into our lives include:
  - caring for others
  - charity (time and materially), and
  - showing compassion, empathy and support.
- In short, strong interpersonal relationships and high rates of pro-social behaviour have a buffering effect on the negative impact of stress on health across all domains.

STEP 3:
SHUT IT DOWN

We now have it on good authority that changing our perception of stress and engaging in pro-social activities during periods of stress can significantly mitigate the negative effects of stress. Of equal importance is the ability to shut down the stress response as soon as it is not required. This is becoming increasingly more challenging in this day and age.

In addition to the faster pace of life now, possible explanations for the ever-increasing levels of stress in our lives are:

- higher expectations from others and of ourselves
- greater competition in all areas of life
- higher levels of intolerance and impatience within society
- constant stimuli
- weakened relationships and connections with others

Fortunately, science has discovered the 'off button'. All we need to do is learn the skills to access this failsafe.

THE VAGUS NERVE

The vagus nerve is an important factor in stress resilience. We already know that stress in short bursts can be highly beneficial, but that relentless activation of the stress response exhausts all the systems of the body, which leads to poor health, lowered functionality and even premature mortality.

The ability to rapidly shut down the stress response and restore biological balance is the cornerstone of stress resilience.

Under healthy circumstances, the stress response will shut itself down via a negative feedback loop once the stressor has dissipated. A negative feedback loop simply means that higher concentrations of stress hormones result in the brain shutting down the stimulus to produce them. However, if stress is chronic and too severe, the body eventually becomes desensitised and the brain is unable to turn off the stress axis. This exposes the brain to excess cortisol and other stress hormones, which further inflict damage and dysregulation[1] of physical and psychological processes.

The critical issue here is that the longer one has been stressed, the more difficult it is to shut down the stress axis. Also, the fact that we get stressed so often is becoming a major health risk. In this and similar situations, deliberate activation of the vagus nerve is one possible way to restore biological balance.

The vagus nerve is one of the longest and most influential nerves in the body. It exits the skull just behind the ears and descends vertically along the front of the throat through the chest cavity and continues down into the abdomen. It is the direct interface between the brain and key organs and systems of the body, most notably the heart, lungs and digestive tract. This so-called wandering nerve operates far below the level of our conscious minds. Although its primary role is synchronicity between the body and the brain, its best-recognised attribute is that of calming the body following the fight-or-flight state induced by adrenalin.

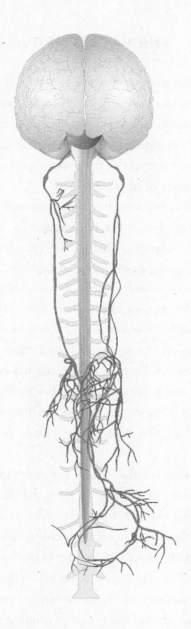

Figure 9 The pathway of the vagus nerve

This is not to say that the vagus nerve is not able to activate the stress axis. Numerous research papers have reliably shown that in both human and animal models vagal stimulation[2] has strong anti-inflammatory effects, some of which are through the release of cortisol (51). However, the mechanism of stress axis stimulation is vastly different. According to neuropharmacologist Dr Kelly Olson (52), the vagus nerve's influence on the stress axis is derived from a real disturbance in physiological systems, such as exercise, fever and pain, in which it confers direct and immediate benefit to the body, without damaging effects. More commonly, the stress axis is activated through the anticipation of a threat or challenge to biological equilibrium. Simply put, the cortisol release that occurs by means of the vagus nerve is due to a real, tangible threat to the system that requires immediate action. More typically, cortisol is released in anticipation of a threat or in response to psychological influences.

Medical researchers have long known that the stronger your vagal tone,[3] the quicker the body can normalise itself following a perceived threat or stressful event; this includes an optimal uptake of oxytocin within the brain. This may explain why some people are seemingly immune to chronic stress, while others become overwhelmed and ill from even the slightest upset. Research shows that poor vagal tone is associated with a compromised biological state, culminating in significant immune dysregulation and chronic inflammation.

Research pioneered largely by Kevin Tracey, a world-renowned professor of Neurosurgery and Molecular Medicine, has shown the vagus nerve to be a master controller of inflammation and immune behaviours within the body, not just through the stress axis and cortisol, but through two additional pathways: the cholinergic anti-inflammatory pathway and the splenic sympathetic anti-inflammatory pathway.

According to Tracey, the vagus nerve interfaces with the spleen signalling specialised immune cells (T-cells) to release acetylcholine,[4] which stimulates cells called macrophages[5] to shut down the production of a key pro-inflammatory chemical known as TNF[6] (53). Dysregulation of TNF is associated with numerous stress-related diseases, including dementia, Alzheimer's, depression, anxiety, cancer, rheumatoid arthritis and inflammatory disorders of the digestive system. When there is good vagal tone and the vagus nerve is frequently stimulated through various activities and exercise, TNF is properly moderated, which promotes and protects health.

In recent years, there has been a wave of research showing the effectiveness of vagal stimulation in a variety of clinical settings. A 2016 multinational study (54) showed how vagus nerve activation could successfully treat rheumatoid arthritis.

Recently, French researchers discovered that vagus nerve stimulation could be used to successfully manage Crohn's disease[7] and even result in remission (55). An extensive 25-year review of the literature on vagus nerve stimulation and neurological health outcomes (56) showed that vagus nerve stimulation can successfully alleviate the symptoms of Alzheimer's disease as well as enhance memory and cognition in healthy individuals.

Vagal tone also appears to play a role in promoting balance in stress hormone levels and stress responses. In 2014, a large team of French researchers published an article on the relationship between vagal tone, cortisol, adrenalin, inflammatory cells and digestive diseases (57). The study involved 73 participants who were divided into three groups: a healthy control group, a group suffering from Crohn's disease and a group diagnosed with irritable bowel syndrome (IBS).

Salivary cortisol was measured the day before the experiment. On the day of the experiment, subjects completed questionnaires for anxiety (State-Trait Anxiety Inventory) and depressive symptoms (Center for Epidemiologic Studies Depression Scale). The researchers performed extensive examinations on all the participants, including salivary cortisol at various intervals throughout the day and blood samples to assess cortisol, adrenalin, noradrenalin and inflammatory markers. Additionally, all subjects were subjected to an electrocardiogram to assess vagal tone and integrity.

The findings revealed that those in the control group with the highest vagal tone showed the lowest cortisol levels towards the end of the day, which reflects optimal balance in daily biological rhythms. Furthermore, there was an inverse relationship between vagal tone and circulating adrenalin in the IBS patients. The Crohn's disease patients showed an inverse association between vagal tone and level of inflammation.

The message that can be extracted from this data is that vagal tone and function translate into biological balance. In healthy subjects, biological rhythms are maximised. In IBS patients, adrenalin is blunted thereby protecting the intestines from further reductions in blood supply and motility compromise. Lastly, in Crohn's patients, where inflammation is a driving force in the intestinal pathology, inflammation is reduced.

Knowing the immense value that the vagus nerve holds in balancing the body's reactions during periods of chronic stress, in addition to the promotion of organ and hormonal health, what can we do to ensure proper tone and function?

An analogy I often use is that of stretching after sport or exercise. Why do we stretch? Most of the time it's unpleasant, not to mention time-consuming. But it does make us feel better.

The principal reason that we stretch is to restore tired muscles to their normal resting length. In this way, the strains of exercise are reduced and the benefits enhanced. In the same way, activation of the vagus nerve following stressful periods rapidly brings our bodies and minds back to a state of balance, reducing the potential for adverse effects.

Fortunately, there are many activities and practices that can increase the activity of the vagus nerve and even improve its tone.

I have selected a handful of the more effective modalities that can be included in a weekly schedule during periods of stress. These are:

- visceral manipulation
- massage therapy

- controlled breathing exercises
- swimming
- cold water facial immersion
- yoga
- meditation, and
- music.

Caution: Anyone with a history of reflex syncope – a dysfunction of the heart rate and blood pressure regulating mechanisms – should not participate in these activities without prior clearance from their doctor.

Visceral manipulation

Visceral manipulation, sometimes referred to as visceral osteopathy, is fast becoming one of the most valued and sought-after practices within conservative healthcare. The founder, Jean Pierre Barral, was cited by *TIME* magazine as one of the top innovators to watch within the medical space. Remarkably, visceral manipulation practitioners are able to interface directly and indirectly with the vagus nerve at various locations throughout the body, profoundly influencing biological balance as well as immune function.

TIME AND TIME AGAIN, I have had patients arrive at my rooms in a state of anxiety, experiencing pain in almost every region of their body and completely exhausted from the pressures and challenges they face in day-to-day life. Before I even begin to address regional pain issues, I get them to lie on the table and then I treat the vagus nerve as it exits the skull, and some of its peripheral branches. Within a few minutes the patients relax into a normalised state. Their pain subsides, their anxieties disappear and they often fall asleep. The reason is that the stress axis has been shut down through the vagal intervention. This is like pressing a stress 'off button'.

Another advantage of visceral manipulation is that it can restore normal mobility and functionality to our internal organs, glands and even deep nerve pathways. This is relevant as research shows that chronic stress is associated with significant disruptions in organ and glandular motility[8] as well as increased tension in the muscular, skeletal and nervous systems. The issue is that this disrupted physical state then sets off the stress axis leading to increased cortisol and adrenalin output, thereby perpetuating a vicious and unrelenting cycle.

Furthermore, not only can compromise to organ motility trigger the stress axis, so can abnormal tension in muscular, skeletal and nervous systems. The reason lies in part with a chain of nerves that runs down the spinal column (from T1 to L3). This chain of stimulatory nerves, known as the sympathetic trunk, can heighten activity in the adrenal glands, as well as many other biological systems. As you may recall, the adrenal glands and the sympathetic trunk form the basis of the working arm of the fight-or-flight response. Spinal immobility or misalignment in this area together with elevated muscular tension have also been shown to trigger the stress axis causing an even greater degree of physical and mental strain.

This is why visceral manipulation practitioners are so unique and are such an invaluable resource during periods of chronic stress. They not only have the skill set to directly stimulate the vagus nerve, they also have the ability to mobilise organs and glands, manipulate the spinal column, release muscular tension, as well as manually desensitise the sympathetic nervous system. Without question, this collective constitutes one of the most comprehensive positive corrections of the stress response. This is why I believe that very few other modalities can offer comparable benefits.

My advice is to have a weekly or bimonthly session with a visceral manipulation specialist during periods of chronic stress. When life is more settled, a monthly check-up is the way forward.

To find a practitioner near you, visit the Barral Institute website.

Massage therapy

In a 2014 study (58), Canadian researchers discovered that light massage on the carotid artery (located near the front of the throat) could stimulate the vagus nerve to such an extent that it could suppress seizures in people who were predisposed to them.

Full-body massage also has a profound effect on vagal activity. Over the last decade, researchers at the University of Miami School of Medicine have published a series of studies investigating the effects of moderate pressure massage and its relationship to vagus nerve activity (59).

Although the studies focused primarily on weight gain in pre-term infants, the data was extremely insightful and can be useful in the management of chronic stress across all age groups. The research team discovered that stimulation of pressure receptors in the muscular and skeletal system through massage therapy dramatically increased vagus nerve activity. More importantly, this vagal activation increased gastric motility by 49%, which resulted in enhanced nutrient absorption.

This is particularly relevant in terms of chronic stress because stress hormones have a dramatic impact on digestive integrity. Increased gastric acid secretion, reduced motility, an underproduction of digestive enzymes and a significant reduction in blood supply typically accompany elevated stress hormone levels. Any measure that can restore regional integrity needs to be a serious consideration.

Additionally, the researchers found that vagal stimulation through massage therapy positively altered the infant's hormonal levels to promote enhanced growth and physiological development.

Although there are several published studies on the relationship between massage and increased vagal activity, more research needs to be done to provide exact prescriptions encompassing specific regions, the degree of pressure, and the duration and frequency of treatment.

Another well-researched benefit of massage in the treatment of chronic stress is the effect it has on stress hormones and neurochemicals. In 2005, the *International Journal of Neuroscience* (60) published a review on the effects of massage therapy. The analysis included studies on depression, pain syndromes, autoimmune conditions and chronic stress in a variety of life areas. The data showed that regular massage was associated with an average overall reduction in cortisol levels of 31%.

This review also highlighted positive changes in levels of key neurochemicals responsible for emotional and cognitive integrity. According to the research team, regular massage resulted in serotonin[9] increases of as much as 28%. Moreover, the neurotransmitter[10] associated with attention, learning and memory known as dopamine[11] showed an average rise of 31%.

Combined, these studies suggest that massage therapy during periods of chronic stress has stress-alleviating effects through decreased cortisol, and positive cognitive and behavioural effects due to increased serotonin and dopamine.

I suggest a weekly massage session during periods of intense or acute stress. I also recommend lighter or moderate pressures to avoid evoking pain and inflammation. It is important to remember that the primary reason for a massage session is to restore biological balance, which includes better organ mobility and function, as well as reduced cortisol and improved neurochemical balance. A massage session is not necessarily for pain management; it would be advisable to consult with your doctor or a physical therapist for this.

Controlled breathing exercises

Numerous studies have shown that slow, controlled breathing exercises[12] increase vagal tone and parasympathetic activity, which result in a dramatic reduction in adrenalin and cortisol levels. Slow, deliberate breathing activates the vagus nerve through more than one pathway, making it highly effective in the management of both short and more sustained stress reactions.

As a general rule, whenever an activity, such as controlled breathing exercises, is able to promote biological change through numerous channels, its value is immense.

One of the mechanisms by which controlled breathing influences the vagus nerve is by stimulating greater sensitivity in cells called baroreceptors. Baroreceptors are super-specialised pressure gauges that are strategically located in arterial walls[13] to detect rises in blood pressure.

Baroreceptors respond to the pressure-induced stretching of the blood vessels in which they are found. This action is known as baroreflex. They communicate this information through the vagus nerve to the brain in order to promote biological stability and functionality. The brain then uses the vagus nerve to slow heart rate and lower blood pressure.

Baroreceptor sensitivity and the baroreflex are at the forefront of cardiovascular health. Information coming from these receptors results in a vagus-mediated reduction in both heart rate and blood pressure.

According to an article published in the journal *Frontiers in Psychology* (61), controlled breathing exercises are a natural stimulus and strengthening mechanism for baroreceptors, which creates heightened awareness in the cardiovascular system. Most importantly, controlled breathing exercises result in an improved capacity to correct the abnormal biological states that typically accompany chronic stress.

In case you're wondering how the cardiovascular system can be said to have 'heightened awareness', consider that all biological systems have complex feedback mechanisms that rely on highly specialised sensors to communicate with the brain or even directly with other organs. Baroceptors are a perfect example of this. What is interesting about the cardiovascular system (of which baroreceptors are a part) is the degree of interaction and influence over other biological systems, including our brain. For example, the heart contains over 40 000 highly specialised nerve cells that have a major influence on the functionality of numerous regions of our brain and even the spinal chord. What's incredible is that the performance of these specialised cells and sensors can be enhanced. Within the context of baroreceptors, regular rather than sporadic controlled breathing exercises strengthen the baroreflex to such an extent that studies show [62] it to be effective in the management of high blood pressure [hypertension], a common health issue attributed to chronic stress. The baroreflex also directly interfaces with the amygdala. This feedback system creates greater emotional stability, which may be why research is showing that controlled breathing exercises are effective in treating depression and anxiety disorders [61].

Yet another way in which controlled breathing exercises inhibit the stress axis is through stimulation of vagal branches found just below the diaphragm. High amplitude expansion and contraction of the ribcage stimulates these vagal connections to the brain and has been shown to have a direct effect on mood regulation. According to an article entitled *"Neuroanatomy of visceral nociception: vagal and splanchnic afferent"*, vagal nerve branches in this region communicate directly with no fewer than five major regions of the brain, including the emotional and memory centres (63).

Furthermore, deep breathing exercises increase vagal activity by elongating lung tissue. Our lungs are infiltrated with tiny stretch receptors known as mechanoreceptors. When activated through large inspirations or even passive stretching (visceral manipulation) the vagus nerve is triggered, which then lowers both heart and respiratory rate.

Finally, not only are the peripheral feedback systems[14] engaged and stimulated through controlled breathing exercises, they can also achieve an increase in vagal output (strength) and overall tone, according to Dr Paul Lehrer, a professor of Occupational Medicine at Rutgers University.

Selecting a breathing technique can be a little challenging, considering there are so many to choose from. The durations of inhalation, holds and exhalation have been the subject of intense debate amongst breathing practitioners and scientists. According to a 2013 study (64), many of these techniques, regardless of the rhythms, elicit very similar biological outcomes provided they stay in a range of 5 to 6 breaths per minute. In 2014, the *International Journal of Psychopharmacology* published a study on how differences in breathing patterns and rhythms impact on vagus nerve activity (65). The study involved 47 healthy participants who performed either 6 breaths per minute or 5.5 breaths per minute for a period of 12 minutes. The effects of the two different breathing rates were evaluated, as well as different inhalation and exhalation patterns. Five-count inhalations and 5-count exhalations (5:5) were compared to 4-count inhalations and 6-count exhalations (4:6). In total, four different breathing combinations were compared with spontaneous breathing (12 to 18 breaths per minute) and vagal responsiveness. The conclusion of the study was that the greatest vagal activation and stimulus occurred with 5.5 breaths per minute in a 5:5 ratio.

Practical application

Find a quiet place where you won't be interrupted. You can either sit upright or be lying down before sleep. Slow your breathing rate down to 5 or 6 breaths per minute. Spend equal time on inhalation and exhalation. The goal is to build up to breathing this way for 10 to 12 minutes. Focusing on breathing this way for such a long time may be a bit challenging in the beginning. So start with 3 to 4 minutes before bed for a few days, then add a minute to the process each day until you reach 12 minutes. It is an incredible way to end the day!

Swimming

FOR YEARS MY PERSONAL CHOICES FOR physical exercise included tennis, running, sports agility and weight training. In 2014, while working at the French Open tennis tournament, I decided to do an indoor speed and agility session before the day started.

It was difficult to watch all those super-agile athletes without wanting to be part of the action.

These types of training sessions involved running between cones; jumps, sprints and a variety of other tennis and sports movement simulations; and have become a personal favourite.

At about 6 am one morning, after a 30-minute walk from my apartment, I arrived at the indoor training venue only to realise that I didn't have my tennis shoes[15] with me. Having no time to go back to the apartment, I decided to perform the training session in normal trainers – something I would never condone with my patients due to the high risk of sustaining knee or ankle injuries. Big mistake. About 30 minutes into the session, during an abrupt change of direction, I felt a sharp pain in my right knee, which I ignored at the time. I managed to finish the session thanks to raised adrenalin and the opioids that result from intense exercise. However, within an hour, walking became very uncomfortable, and a flight of stairs was almost impossible.

The region of my knee that I injured was the patella tendon, just below the kneecap. I realised that I had sustained a micro-rupture, which is notoriously non-responsive to treatment. As soon as I had the opportunity to receive treatment, I did. I had some of my colleagues work on me for months with little to no change in outcome. Not unexpected, though.

Frustrated with not being able to play tennis, run or perform leg exercises, I decided to take up swimming as a means of maintaining aerobic fitness. I had swum a little as a child but had not swum any appreciable distance for decades. My first swimming session involved around 500 metres, which felt like I had run a marathon – twice! My lungs burned, my muscles ached, and I was extremely embarrassed by my lack of efficiency and coordination. Since tennis and running were out of the question, I had no option but to persevere.

After the initial swimming experience, I realised I needed a technique coach. Fortunately, the gym I belong to has a great swimming instructor, Simon. The first three sessions were horrible, not because of Simon's instruction, but because of my inability to manage my rate of breathing. Incidentally, this is a major factor in the dysregulation of the stress response. I lacked swimming fitness to such a degree that the lessons actually made me stressed.

Perseverance paid off and over time I improved measurably, able to swim distances of 2 to 3 kilometres in a session and, believe it or not, I began thoroughly enjoying the experience.

Surprisingly, it wasn't the gains in fitness or the feeling of accomplishment that motivated me to continue swimming once my knee had recovered,[16] it was the prevailing sense of calm and tranquillity that followed the swimming sessions. I had never experienced this through exercise before.

Additionally, my overall stress levels began to decline, and management of acute stress improved; my reactivity to challenging situations became more moderated. However, what piqued my interest was an unknown variable, which happened to be a biological trend that followed specific drills in the pool. When I performed drills that involved underwater swimming for more than 10 to 15 seconds, the post-session stress-reduction effects were profoundly amplified. I needed to understand why this was, so I began researching the biological mechanisms behind the stress-moderating effect of swimming, specifically underwater swimming. What I was about to find out was that swimming has the potential to be one of the greatest tools in stress management.

The reasons that swimming, specifically underwater swimming, is so beneficial are multifactorial.[17] It all starts with the survival reaction known as the **diving reflex**. This vagal-mediated safety reflex overrides all biological states and occurs in response to water submersion and our corresponding breath-holding. In simple terms, survival always takes precedence. No matter what biological state you are in, when you submerge yourself in water, the brain's first response is to stop breathing and slow down your biological processes.

Scientists have found the diving reflex to be particularly strong in infants between four and twelve months old. However, as in many areas of our health and functionality, with advancing age this important reflex weakens and will require retraining and frequent stimulus to remain effective. This explains why I found the first few swimming sessions so challenging in terms of regulating my breathing.

While swimming and submergence in water are strong activators of the vagus nerve and result in a corresponding reduction in heart rate by 10–25%, the biological process is very complex. According to a 2009 article (66), submergence in water initially triggers a fight-or-flight reaction for a few seconds. This means that there is a slight rise in arterial pressure as blood and lung oxygen stores are preferentially redistributed to the heart and the brain. Many other biological shifts take place, including the release of red blood cells from the spleen. We have all experienced that 'gasp' moment when diving into a pool or submerging our head in cool water.

Following this alarm state, there is a strong vagal presence and corresponding calming of your biological state via two distinct mechanisms. The first is through baroreflex activation from the rise in blood pressure, and the second is from chemical receptor stimulation that occurs as oxygen levels decline during the latter part of a breath-hold.

Research has shown that there are many additional factors that can intensify the vagal response and positive biological shifts, especially the combination of movement and breath-holding under water. A study on vagal activation in response to water submersion (67) showed that swimming underwater can reduce heart rate by more than 50% within less than 30 seconds, which is greater than the effect seen in simple submergence.

Furthermore, vagal activity is amplified if the water is cool. The reason for this is that cold water contact[18] in and around the forehead, eyes and mouth is a strong stimulus for the fifth cranial nerve, the trigeminal nerve, which activates the vagus nerve. As you can see, the parasympathetic nervous system is activated via several different pathways that include pressure receptors, oxygen and gas receptors, and nerve centres in the face. This said, the aerobic nature of swimming, combined with the rhythmic breathing that accompanies this activity adds an additional dimension to the stress-reduction equation.

Although many forms of exercise offer enormous value in chronic stress management and health outcomes, research shows that swimming offers some of the greatest value in this space.

In 2008, Nancy Chase and a team of researchers at the University of South Carolina published a study on all-cause mortality risk comparing swimmers, runners, walkers and sedentary men (68). A total of 40 547 men between the ages of 20 and 90 were examined over an average period of 13 years.

A comprehensive multi-variable analysis was performed on the group to ensure the results were not corrupted by any additional factors. This included age (in years), body mass index (BMI), smoking status (current smoker or not), weekly alcohol intake (≥5 drinks or none), medical conditions (including cardiovascular disease, hypertension, diabetes, or hypercholesterolaemia), as well as a family medical history.

There were 3 386 deaths during the extensive period of observation. After adjustments were made for age, BMI, smoking status, alcohol intake, and family history of cardiovascular disease, swimmers had the lowest risk of premature death. So much so that compared with those who were sedentary there was a 53% lower risk of premature mortality in the thirteen-year follow-up. It may not come as a surprise that swimming offers substantial health returns when compared with inactivity. However, where the results of the study were unexpected is that swimming was associated with the lowest risk of premature mortality when compared with walking and running, which reduced the risk by 50% and 49% respectively.

The researchers investigated possible mechanisms to explain why swimmers had such low rates of mortality when compared with the other groups. It was found that swimmers had significantly better health profiles, including a lower resting rate and lower total cholesterol, triglycerides, fasting blood glucose, as well as other positive health markers when compared to sedentary men. This was certainly not unexpected. They also had lower resting heart rates, lower total cholesterol and triglyceride levels when compared with walkers – again, not surprising. However, what was surprising was the fact that the swimmers and runners had similar profiles, yet swimmers had a significantly lower risk of mortality. The only explanation is possibly higher vagal tone or a greater degree of vagus nerve activation through to various pathways. However, before policy recommendations can be made, more research needs to be done to confirm these findings and properly clarify the unknown variables.

> During periods of intense or chronic stress, try to get to a swimming pool or any other place where you can swim safely. It doesn't matter whether you swim lengths or merely wade, as long as you get your head under the water and enjoy the experience.

Practical application

Try to incorporate some form of swimming into a weekly routine during periods of high stress. The frequency, intensity and duration are dependent on your inherent fitness levels, access to aquatic facilities and time availability. I would recommend one to three sessions a week when stress levels are high, specifically towards the end of the day.

As with many modalities in the health space, moderation appears to offer the greatest returns. This is no different with vagal tone, biological balance and their relationship to swimming. In 2011, Brazilian researchers (69) investigated the influence of the duration of physical training sessions on vagal tone, specifically cardiac autonomic[19] adaptations. The study divided lab rats into four groups: one sedentary group and three training groups subjected to swimming for 15, 30 and 60 minutes a day for a period of 10 weeks. All three training groups showed positive cardiovascular adaptations, but only the 30- and 60-minute swimming groups showed an increase in vagal tone relative to the sedentary group. Interestingly, when the 30- and 60-minute swimming sessions were compared, it wasn't the longer session, but the shorter of the two sessions that promoted superior results.

The message from this study reinforces the notion that moderation is necessary to achieve optimal health, especially in the context of chronic stress management.

Cold facial immersion

Have you ever wondered why there have been periods in your life when you feel out of balance, whether emotionally or physically, and your instinctive response was to splash cold water on your face, have a cold shower or dive into a cold pool? What we intuitively know is that cold water facial immersion promotes a sense of calm and triggers a greater degree of biological balance.

Over the last two decades numerous studies have appeared in the literature (70, 71) showing that cold exposure to the face, particularly with water, is a potent trigger in vagus nerve activity. In fact, this effect is so powerful that cold water facial immersion for one to three minutes is often used by scientists as a functional assessment of vagus nerve integrity. Cold water facial immersion mimics many of the biological effects of the diving reflex; however, not through internal pressure or chemical receptors, but through the trigeminal nerve instead.

Although often compared to the diving reflex, stimulation of this facial nerve is an independent reflex known as the trigeminal cardiac reflex. It is easy to confuse the two as swimming in ice-cold water would activate the trigeminal cardiac reflex as well as the diving reflex.

In 2015, a research article comparing the diving and trigeminal cardiac reflexes was published in the *Archives of Medical Science* (72). The researchers identified several similarities, but the trigeminal cardiac reflex had distinct advantages that apply to reducing the stress response. Stimulation of the trigeminal cardiac reflex is a strong vagal activator that results not only in a rapid reduction in heart rate, but also in reduced blood pressure, and importantly, increased visceral motility.

Considering that acute and chronic stress are associated with elevated heart rate, elevated blood pressure and reduced organ movement, in many respects this reflex is diametrically opposed to the stress axis and offers biological protection under a variety of challenging conditions. The powerful effects of this reflex in humans were first described by Swiss researchers in the *Journal of Neurosurgery* (73) almost two decades ago. The neurosurgeons pointed out that this reflex is characterised by a 20% drop in blood pressure and heart rate levels below 60 beats per minute (bpm).

Interestingly, many forms of therapy, such as osteopathy, cranial sacral[20] therapy, EFT[21] tapping, head massage, acupressure and acupuncture successfully use this reflex to obtain a state of biological balance and improved health. Although the trigeminal cardiac reflex is a physiological oxygen-conserving reflex, when triggered it first increases blood to the brain. This regional elevation of blood flow without accompanying changes in the local metabolic use of oxygen or glucose provides oxygen to the brain in a highly efficient manner, promoting better functionality.

The relationship between cold water facial immersion and the stress axis was properly explored in a 2011 study published in *Psychophysiology* (74). The study by Swiss and Canadian researchers was able to identify that not only does cold water facial immersion lower heart rate and blood pressure and improve organ functionality, it also impacts mood and stress hormone profiles.

The study involved 33 participants who completed a simulated stress task that induced a rise in cortisol, heart rate and blood pressure, and a negative emotional state. This certainly wouldn't be a challenge in this day and age! Once the participants were measurably stressed, they were required to wear a face pack that was only 1°C/34°F for approximately 2 minutes. The face pack had openings for the eyes and nose. Incredibly, within less than 30 seconds the participants' heart rates started to slow as the stress axis began shutting down. The study also provided two important insights relating to stress hormones and vagal tone:

1 Cortisol elevations in response to stress are not immediate, they are delayed. Typically, the elevation of cortisol in response to stress begins about 15 minutes after the event, peaks at about 40 minutes, and does not return to baseline until well after 80 minutes.

2. Participants who showed greater vagal tone, as measured by EEG, experienced an 18% reduction in cortisol spikes. Higher vagal tone was also associated with less emotional reactivity to stress, and enhanced mood states when compared with the rest of the group.

The more you stimulate the vagus nerve with breathing exercises, swimming, cold facial immersion, osteopathy, massage and other similar practices, the greater your resilience will be during emotionally and physically stressful events. The same is true for managing chronic stress.

Cold water facial immersion certainly provides a quick and easy solution to managing stressful situations in a variety of settings. However, a simple splash of cold water in the office bathroom may not be enough to achieve proper correction of the stress axis. According to medical experts from the Cleveland Clinic's Center for Integrative Medicine, an actual facial submersion may be necessary. Fortunately, water temperatures need not be 1°C/34°F, but rather a more pleasant 10°C/50°F to 11°C/52°F. Japanese researchers (70) found that the greatest vagal responses were achieved by facial submergence in water that was 4°C/39°F for periods of around 30 seconds.

Lastly, if you don't want to be caught with your head submerged in a basin of cold water at work, try to get to the gym or home at lunchtime for a cold swim, shower or bath. The benefit will be well worth the time and effort.

Another easy option is to purchase a cold face pack, typically used to manage puffiness and facial inflammation, which can be easily found online. You can keep these in the fridge and place them on your face for 1–3 minutes at a time.

Yoga

The practice of yoga has been growing in popularity in recent years – and with good reason. In addition to the numerous benefits attributed to yoga such as increased flexibility, balance, coordination and strength, research shows that yoga may be successful in managing the stress axis and promoting stress resilience.

In 2016, Australian researchers published an extensive meta-analysis on the relationship between yoga practice and vagal tone, as measured by heart rate variability[22] (75). Unlike many other aspects in life, changeability within this context actually provides a greater indication of heath and stress resilience across numerous domains.

The meta-analysis involved 2 358 participants drawn from 59 studies. Although many of the studies were poorly designed and had small sample groups, 15 studies were randomised control trials, of which some were highly rated according to the Oxford Quality Scoring System.

The review evaluated numerous variables, including the frequency and duration of yoga practice, the participants' experience and their respective health profiles. Because yoga practice is highly diverse, it is a challenge to properly assess yoga and health outcomes. Yoga encompasses a range of activities, such as:

- physical postures and exercises to promote strength and flexibility
- breathing exercises to enhance respiratory functioning
- deep relaxation techniques to cultivate the ability to mentally and physiologically release tension and stress
- meditation/mindfulness practices to enhance mind-body awareness and improve attention and emotion regulation skills.

Diversity of practice notwithstanding, the researchers concluded that there is considerable evidence that yoga increases vagal activity during practice, which translates to improved biological integrity and stress resilience. More importantly, the review found that regular yoga practitioners have increased vagal tone at rest when compared with non-yoga practitioners.

There have been numerous reviews by researchers from around the world on the effects of yoga as an alternative and complementary approach to managing chronic stress (76, 77). Many of these reviews support the practice of yoga in stress management; however, they raise concerns about study designs, length, sample size, standardisation of practice, and variability in outcomes. Therefore, the authors suggest that the findings should be interpreted with caution because further investigation is warranted.

The *Journal of Evidence-Based Complementary and Alternative Medicine* recently published a pilot study on the effects of classroom yoga on behaviour and stress hormone levels in adolescents (78).

The study was run by a large team, which included researchers from both Harvard and Yale universities and involved two classrooms of 2nd and 3rd grade[23] scholars. In total, 36 scholars participated in the 10-week study, which involved only 30 minutes of yoga practice every week. The outcome of the study was interesting in that the younger and older groups responded somewhat differently. Whereas the 3rd graders showed no change in cortisol, the 2nd graders had a more than 30% reduction in baseline cortisol values over the 10-week period. The teacher ratings for the 2nd graders revealed improvements in:

- social interaction with classmates
- attention span
- ability to concentrate on work
- ability to stay on task
- academic performance
- ability to deal with stress/anxiety, and
- confidence/self-esteem and overall mood.

The 3rd graders did not reveal the same behavioural changes, but did show perceived improvements in creativity, ability to control behaviour, and ability to manage anger. Considering that these responses were from limited practice of just 30 minutes a week, this is quite remarkable.

Interestingly, both groups responded favourably in terms of lowered cortisol responses to attention- and focus-based tests. Simply put, over the 10-week period both the 2nd and 3rd graders showed a blunted cortisol response to the simulated stress. These results support prior research suggesting that yoga may increase mental health, positive behaviours, and well-being in children and adolescents.

In 2013, Indian researchers published a study on the cortisol-lowering and antidepressant effects of regular yoga practice (79). The study highlighted the relationship between depression, excessive cortisol production and overactivation of the stress axis. This bidirectional relationship between stress and depression is extremely important because both are highly prevalent in today's society and pose a significant challenge to healthcare systems, the corporate environment and the economy as a whole.

The three-month study divided 58 depressed participants into three groups: group 1 received antidepressant medication; group 2 received yoga sessions; group 3 received both yoga sessions and antidepressant medication. A separate control group of 18 participants was also included.

Both cortisol levels and depression[24] were assessed prior to treatment and at the end of the study.

Adherence to treatment was operationally defined as doing 50 or more yoga sessions in a three-month period and/or taking medication for at least two months.

What the researchers found was that the depressed participants had markedly higher cortisol levels than the controls (>30%), confirming a direct correlation between cortisol levels and depression. Over the three-month study period, all three groups showed improvements in depression ratings. However, not all groups showed reductions in cortisol levels. In all patients who practised yoga, with or without medication, the changes in cortisol levels were significant (±20%). However, those who only received medication did not show the same stabilisation in the stress axis, and in some cases, cortisol levels were actually significantly higher following treatment.

The study also showed that the relationship between reduced cortisol and lowered depression was most apparent in the yoga-only treatment group. The researchers propose numerous mechanisms through which these effects take place, highlighting an increase in vagal tone, a reduction in circulating adrenalin, elevated concentrations of molecules that enhance brain structure and function, as well as regional shifts in brain activation.

This study confirmed the benefits of yoga in depressed individuals with high stress hormone profiles. The question is how would yoga benefit healthy individuals subjected to significant amounts of stress due to high professional demands and an unpredictable working environment?

The *International Journal of Research in Medical Sciences* recently published a study on the effects of yoga on 40 medical students between the ages of 18 and 25 (80). The group was divided into two, with 20 subjects in a yoga group and 20 subjects in a control group. Morning saliva samples were collected from all participants to measure and compare cortisol levels over the three-month period.

From the outset, both groups had similar cortisol levels; however this was not the case following the three-month study. The control group showed no statistical difference in cortisol levels over the study period. The group practising yoga for an hour every day showed an over 40% reduction in cortisol, indicating lower overall stress profiles.

The authors suggest that the dramatic reduction in cortisol over three months was largely due to increases in vagal tone. They also proposed that the varying postures enhance circulation to vital organs, which promotes better neurological and hormonal balance and integrity.

The authors conclude that yoga may be as effective, if not more so, than any other non-pharmacological therapy for improving a variety of health-related disorders.

The true reason that yoga practice can manage stress lies in the combination of activities that encompass physically demanding postures, controlled breathing exercises and various forms of meditation. While each activity promotes health and stress resilience, the collective effect is nothing short of remarkable.

If you're planning to take up yoga and you have health or orthopaedic issues, it is advisable that you consult with your doctor to get medical clearance. It would also be advantageous initially to have personal instruction either in a small group or individually to reinforce technique as well as some of the finer details of the practice. Although daily practice might not be practical for many people, two or three sessions a week would be of enormous value in terms of stress management and resilience.

Meditation

Meditation has become increasingly popular in recent years. Perhaps the appeal is that it offers a temporary escape from the ever-present chaos of daily life. Or the attraction may be that it is one of the oldest proven methods of managing stress and promoting health.

Although it has been widely practised in various parts of the Middle East and Asia for thousands of years, it is only in recent times that meditation has achieved the recognition it deserves in the rest of the world.

Meditation is a form of mental training that aims to improve your underlying psychological capacities, such as mental clarity and awareness, and emotional self-regulation. There are many forms of meditation ranging from traditional Kabbalistic and Eastern practices, to modern-day programmes focusing on stress, personal growth, and the findings of neuroscience. Meditation may encompass a broad spectrum of complex practices that include the very popular mindfulness meditation, mantra-meditation, yoga, tai chi and even chi gong.

Because meditation practices typically centre around controlled breathing, the majority of these techniques and practices provide a strong vagal stimulus, as discussed in the section on controlled breathing. For this reason, meditation practices apply to both shutting down the stress response (Step 3) and rebuilding and repair (Step 4).

Although there are some inconsistencies in the literature pertaining to the effectiveness of meditation in reducing certain stress-related ailments, the majority of studies show very strong support.

In 2013, researchers from the Center for Mind and Brain at the University of California published a study (81) showing that the practice of mindfulness meditation is associated with lowered cortisol. For the study, 57 people spent three months in a meditation retreat, where they were taught mindful breathing, observation skills, and cultivation of positive mental states, such as compassion. The participants' cortisol levels were measured using a saliva test, and their mindfulness levels were rated on a relevant scale at the start and end of the retreat.

As you might expect, after a three-month retreat of this nature, the researchers found that the participants' mindfulness scores were higher at the end of the retreat than at the beginning. What is interesting is that the researchers found a direct correlation between increases in mindfulness and corresponding decreases in cortisol levels. Moreover, the reductions in cortisol were not consistent throughout the day, but rather were evident at night (which is ideal) showing that the effect of the mindfulness meditation potentiated optimal biological functioning.

> Cortisol has a distinct daily rhythm. To ensure optimal functioning of the body, cortisol is elevated in the morning and tapers off towards the evening. After reaching its lowest point at midnight, the cortisol level begins to rise at around 2 am to 3 am. The cortisol level generally peaks at 8.30 am, which helps us to get going for the day.
>
> Cortisol acts as a secondary messenger between the brain and other systems in the body; it helps orchestrate the timing of the release of many hormones and molecules. Changes in this daily rhythm can be problematic across many areas of health. The primary issue with chronic stress is that cortisol is high later in the day and evening, which is an abnormal occurrence for the body. This not only impacts sleep, but also our ability to wake up, as well as other hormonal and biological processes.

The study was significant in that it identified that increased mindfulness directly correlates to improved functionality of the stress axis. However, the big question is, can we benefit from meditation in a more practical context? In other words, can we benefit without disconnecting from our day-to-day challenges and responsibilities? The science says – yes! A perfect example is a collaborative study performed by researchers from the US and China (82), which showed that just five days of meditation training using a technique called Integrative Body-Mind Training (IBMT) was able to reduce cortisol output in response to acute stress simulations. Additionally, those who practised IBMT also showed lower levels of anxiety, depression, anger and fatigue than the control group.

In 2017, a group of prominent researchers[25] published a paper (83) on mindfulness meditation training on acute stress responses in people who have generalised anxiety disorder.[26]

The study involved 89 participants who were randomly divided into two groups: group 1 took an eight-week mindfulness-based stress reduction course; group 2, the control group, took an eight-week Stress Management Education (SME) course.

The SME course involved general tips on the importance of good nutrition, sleep habits and other relevant wellness topics. Both programmes had similar formats. The main difference was that only Group 1 learned meditative techniques during their course.

Participants underwent the Trier Social Stress Test[27] before and after the course.

During the stress simulation, the research team monitored a range of biological markers in the subjects' stress responses. These markers included ACTH[28] and the inflammatory proteins IL-6 and TNF-α.

When the two groups were compared, Group 2 actually showed slight increases in stress hormones and inflammatory markers on the second test[29] compared with the first. It was speculated that this was caused by anticipatory anxiety knowing that the test would be repeated.

However, the meditation group showed significant declines in all the biological stress markers on the second test, implying that the meditation training had reduced the activity of the stress axis itself.

Although meditation is often used primarily as a means of reducing and managing stress, its greatest value lies in its capacity to enhance brain functionality and structure.

Meditation affects brain morphology[30]

The ways in which meditation practices can change the composition of the brain ultimately form the basis of the effectiveness of meditation in chronic stress management.

In the past decade, there have been numerous studies investigating alterations in brain morphology related to meditation. In a 2014 meta-analysis (84) of 21 neuro-imaging studies that examined some 300 meditation practitioners, researchers found that there were eight regions of the brain that showed distinct morphological changes. These included increases in grey matter volume and concentration, as well as cortical thickness. The regions that controlled awareness, memory, inter-hemispheric communication, and emotional regulation showed the most marked effects. The authors considered these effects to be highly significant.

A team of prominent researchers from the US and Germany, led by Britta Hölzel of Harvard Medical School, published a study investigating the before- and after-effects of Mindfulness-Based Stress Reduction (MBSR) on the characteristics of grey matter (85). MBSR is one of the most widely used mindfulness training programmes and has been reported to produce positive effects on psychological well-being and to ameliorate the symptoms of a number of health disorders.

The study involved a group of 16 participants who were inexperienced in meditation. They underwent extensive neuro-imagery (MRIs) before and after the 8-week programme. Interestingly, the participants reported spending a total of only 22.6 hours engaged in formal homework throughout the study. This works out to an average of only 27 minutes of home meditation practice per day. Changes in grey matter concentrations were investigated using voxel-based morphometry.[31] The results were then compared with a control group of 17 participants.

The brain scans revealed increases in grey matter concentrations within the left hippocampus as well as increases in the posterior cingulate cortex, the temporo-parietal junction, and the cerebellum in the MBSR group when compared with the controls.

Simply put, the results show that less than 30 minutes of MBSR practice a day is associated with positive changes in the regions of the brain involved in learning, memory and emotional regulation. These results are especially significant in that chronic stress is strongly associated with compromise to both brain functionality and structure.

Without going into too much detail, the hippocampus has been shown to shrink in response to chronic stress through a variety of mechanisms. These processes include:

- nerve cell loss due to chronic elevations of cortisol
- glial cell[32] loss
- a stress-induced reduction in proteins that promote nerve cell retention and formation, known as neurotrophins,[33] and
- a stress-induced reduction in the formation of new nerve cells.

Reduced hippocampal size is strongly correlated with depression and other stress-related psychopathologies.

Based on the existing body of research into the relationship between meditation and positive morphological changes in the brain, it is plausible that meditative practices may be one of the most effective therapies in managing the long-term effects of chronic stress, not to mention several mental health issues. It is nothing short of astounding that the regions of the brain that show the greatest degree of improvement through regular meditation practices are the very regions that are the most compromised in response to exposure to chronic stress.

Research has also shown that meditation can have beneficial effects in a number of cognitive domains, including attention, memory, verbal fluency, executive function, processing speed, overall cognitive flexibility and conflict monitoring, and even creativity (86).

Meditation protects the brain from the ageing process

The brain is our most precious resource. Every facet of our lives is influenced by this complex organ. Despite its vital role, it is extremely fragile and is particularly prone to compromise as we age.

According to Ruth Peters at the Imperial College Faculty of Medicine in

London (87), the volume of the brain and/or its weight decline with age at a rate of around 5% per decade from the age of 40. Moreover, the rate of decline increases dramatically with advancing age particularly over the age of 70.

Chronic stress may further amplify this process, progressively and rapidly corroding brain cells and intrinsic blood vessels, together with our cognition.

Nevertheless, there are a few modalities that can combat this biological crisis, one of which is meditation.

In a research article entitled "Forever young(er): potential age-defying effects of long-term meditation on gray matter atrophy" (86) scientists from the University of California and the Australian National University in Canberra were able to identify numerous positive effects of long-term meditation practices on the ageing brain.

The study involved 100 participants, 50 of whom were meditation practitioners. The other 50 formed the control group. The meditators and controls were closely matched in chronological age, ranging from 24 to 77. Meditation experience was variable, and typically ranged between 4 and 46 years. When examining the link between chronological age and whole-brain grey matter, the researchers observed a significant negative correlation in both groups. The trend was that the older the participant, the more significant the decline in brain mass. This reaffirmed findings from other studies that show that ageing causes a considerable decline in brain mass.

However, the slopes of the regression lines were considerably steeper in the controls than in meditators, implying that meditation practices are able to slow down the rate of age-associated brain atrophy. The researchers then turned their attention to focal regions within the brain, specifically those that are susceptible to compromise and shrinkage in response to the ageing process. It should come as no surprise that these were considerably more atrophied in the controls than in the meditators. This pattern echoed the broader grey-matter observations in that the decline of age-sensitive regions was far less prominent in those who meditated regularly.

Although this was certainly one of the larger and more recent studies that involved a diverse group of participants of all ages, there have been several studies on smaller groups of younger subjects that show even greater neuroprotective effects. The implication is that the sooner you start meditating the greater the potential to protect your brain from stress and ageing (87).

For example, in 2007 researchers from Emory University in Atlanta published a study (88) that investigated the effects of Zen meditation[34] on brain integrity. The study involved 26 participants whose average age was 36. Thirteen of the subjects practised Zen meditation regularly and had more than three years' experience. The other 13 subjects were matched controls. While the control subjects displayed the expected negative correlation of both grey matter volume and attentional performance with advancing age, the Zen meditators did not show a significant correlation in either measure with age. In fact, the study estimated the rate of brain mass decline to be in the region of -4.7 ml per year for the control group. Conversely, the Zen meditators actually increased their brain mass by +1.8 ml per year! Interestingly, the region of the brain that benefited the most from Zen meditation was an area known as the putamen. This structure is strongly associated with learning, movement, attention and information processing. According to the authors:

> *These findings suggest that the regular practice of meditation may have neuro-protective effects and reduce the cognitive decline associated with normal aging.*

If you don't already have meditation experience, or are unable to commit a lot of time to this modality, the good news is that it appears that just a few high-quality hours of practice per month are able to induce advantageous neuroplasticity[35] as well as other positive structural changes.

Meditation creates better connectivity within the brain

In 2018, *Frontiers in Systems Neuroscience* published an article entitled "Brief mental training reorganizes large-scale brain networks" (89). The study involved 25 young participants with an average age of 21 who had no prior meditation experience.

The participants received two weeks of IBMT, which involved 30 minutes of practice per session for a total of 10 sessions. All in all, this amounted to 5 hours of meditative training over 14 days. Whole-brain MRI scans were performed on the group to assess patterns of connectivity and brain activity before and after the IBMT training. Incredibly, with only two weeks of meditation training, 60 new functional connections were identified. The regions of the brain that showed the greatest adaptations were those that were involved in cognitive and affective processing, emotion and sleep regulation, as well as coordination, posture and balance.

Insights from neuro-imagery and studies on meditation's effect on brain structure may finally resolve the contentious debate surrounding the possible effectiveness of meditation and related interventions in managing the acute symptoms of stress and improving long-term health outcomes.

Meditation alters brain activity and lowers stress hormone output

Carnegie Mellon University Medical School has been a leader in the study of the brain and behaviour for more than 50 years. It is not surprising that researchers from this prestigious institution may have identified the mechanism by which meditation can positively influence our experience of stress.

David Creswell, a professor of Psychology (90), and his graduate student Emily Lindsay, suggest that mindfulness meditation positively influences health via stress reduction pathways. These pathways allude to the distinctive shifts in brain activity that occur following regular exposure to meditation.

Many scientists believe that this model offers one of the first evidence-based biological accounts of mindfulness training and its relationship to stress reduction. In essence, the model has cracked the code in terms of meditation's ability to reduce and buffer many of the adverse effects of chronic stress.

Creswell's detailed model of how mindfulness meditation is able to change stress processing in the brain was presented in an article published in 2014 in *Current Directions in Psychological Science* (90).

The paper describes how definitive alterations in brain activity induced by mindfulness meditation and related interventions are able to blunt the physiological stress-response, which includes elevated cortisol, adrenalin and inflammatory proteins. The less extreme biological reactions to perceived threats and daily challenges dramatically reduce the corresponding risk of developing stress-related ailments.

In essence, Creswell found that two things happen in response to regular mindfulness meditation:

1. The logical centres[36] of the brain are developed and strengthened, which then overshadow the emotional centres when we encounter stressful situations. This changes our response to the daily challenges we face, making our experience less emotional and more intellectual.
2. The centres in the brain responsible for stress processing become less reactive and more stable when confronted with a stressful situation. In a sense, they become desensitised. Neuro-imaging studies corroborate these finding (91) showing that the amygdala displays alterations in connectivity and structure.

A 2013 study on 155 participants (321) that factored in demographic and individual differences, including age, total grey matter volume and psychopathologies, showed that those with higher dispositional mindfulness[37] showed reductions in size of several stress processing centres, suggesting that more permanent changes may occur from long-term meditation.

Meditation influences our DNA

While mind-body interventions like meditation, yoga and tai chi positively alter brain morphology, reorganise the stress response at a central level, and are able to lower cortisol and adrenalin, the greatest benefit may be related to their influence on genetic behaviours.

Over the past decade, studies investigating gene expression patterns in response to mind-body interventions have begun to appear with increasing frequency. In addition to being an objective measure for evaluating and comparing the effectiveness of meditative practices, the analysis of gene expression changes has considerable scientific value because it reveals the underlying mechanisms of the psychological and physical effects of these ancient modalities.

Scientists and researchers have confirmed that the effects of chronic stress go well beyond primary biological systems, organs and hormones and may result in significant dysfunction within our DNA. We know that chronic stress causes telomere corrosion, resulting in genetic instability and increased cellular ageing. Not only does chronic stress result in structural changes to our DNA, it can also significantly alter genetic behaviours and expression through a process called Conserved Transcriptional Response to Adversity (CTRA).

CTRA is a common molecular pattern that has been reliably found in people exposed to various types of adversities and ongoing life challenges (92). CTRA is largely associated with the up-regulation[38] of the genes that increase inflammation at the cellular level.

Whereas short-lived inflammation is a necessary adaptive response that provides protection from both injury and infections, chronic inflammation is maladaptive because it persists after the physical threat is no longer present. Chronic inflammation is associated with increased risk for some types of cancer, accelerated ageing, cardiovascular diseases, neurodegenerative diseases and psychiatric disorders, Crohn's disease, rheumatoid arthritis and even diabetes.

Yet another surprising characteristic of CTRA is the down-regulation of antiviral and antibody-related genes, which is associated with increased susceptibility to viral infections including Epstein Barr and Herpes Simplex. This would appear counter-intuitive considering that the immune system is in a chronic state of over-activation.

The combination of genetic activity favouring inflammation together with reduced antiviral and antibody activity is becoming viewed as the genetic signature of chronic stress (93).

In 2017, *Frontiers in Immunology* (93) published a review investigating the behavioural characteristics of our genetic material during periods of stress, as well as in response to various forms of meditation practice, notably mindfulness, yoga and tai chi.

The research team from England, The Netherlands and Belgium were particularly interested in the potential changes in gene expression that might occur as a result of mind-body interventions. Moreover, they also explored the possible relationship between suspected molecular changes and chronic stress, as well as their possible role in stress-associated health outcomes.

Following a detailed review of the literature, which included 18 studies involving 846 participants over an 11-year period, the researchers concluded that there is a clearly defined pattern of genetic and molecular changes that reduces the numerous negative health effects associated with stress.

Incredibly, the adversity-induced genetic changes favouring inflammatory states were neutralised by mind-body interventions. According to the authors, 81% of the studies in the meta-analysis that measured the activity of inflammation-related genes and/or NF-κB[39] found a significant inhibitory effect.

What was interesting about the studies in the review was the fact that they were highly variable from both an intervention perspective, and in the way that gene expression was assessed. For example, mind-body interventions varied from individual, seated meditation sessions to different forms of movement therapies in groups. Although 46% of the studies involved a period of six to twelve weeks, some studies were as short as four days, and others as long as four months. The participant profile also varied. Half the studies involved healthy adults, whereas the other half focused on clinical[40] or highly stressed sample groups.

Even with the high degree of variability, the collective data showed extremely positive genetic changes associated with mind-body interventions. Simply put, mind-body therapies lower inflammation and improve antiviral and antibody function.

To give some idea of the scope of genetic adaptations, researchers from various departments at the University of California published a randomised control trial investigating the effects of meditation on those caring for family members with dementia (94). This group was especially relevant as they experience high levels of stress.

The 45 caregivers were randomly assigned to either a twelve-minute per day meditation programme or a twelve-minute per day relaxing music session. Genetic evaluations were performed using white blood cells before and after the eight-week study.

The research showed that short, structured meditation sessions positively altered the behaviour of as many as 68 genes favouring better immune behaviour and lowered inflammation.

Choosing a meditation technique

With so many techniques to choose from, it may be challenging, or even overwhelming, to decide on a suitable one. A quick tour through the research on the effects of meditation practice commonly includes these techniques, which we will cover in this chapter:

- Mindfulness or open monitoring meditation
- Mindfulness-Based Stress Reduction (MBSR)
- Integrative Body-Mind Training (IBMT)
- Zen meditation
- Loving kindness meditation.

My advice is to try various techniques to see which practice resonates the most with you. As with the development of any new skill, it is advisable that you seek expert guidance to ensure that you derive maximum benefit from the experience.

Mindfulness or open monitoring meditation

Mindfulness or open monitoring meditation stems from Eastern meditation practices. This form of meditation emphasises developing an open, accepting attitude, and learning to let go of mental content, neither resisting nor elaborating on anything that surfaces in your awareness.

Mindfulness requires the regulation of attention in order to maintain focus on the immediate experience, such as thoughts, emotions, body posture and physical sensations, as well as the ability to approach these experiences with a level of openness and acceptance.

There are numerous open monitoring techniques, many of which are still an integral part of ancient Eastern meditation practice. There are also several more recent clinical adaptations, such as Mindfulness-Based Stress Reduction[41] (MBSR), Integrative Body-Mind Training (IBMT) and Mindfulness-Based Cognitive Therapy (MBCT).

Mindfulness-Based Stress Reduction (MBSR)

There is a wealth of research supporting the effectiveness of MBSR in chronic stress management in a variety of domains. The standard curriculum is conducted in an 8-week structured group format, which includes weekly 2.5-hour group sessions in addition to a 6-hour day-long retreat. Within this training model participants are taught to observe situations and thoughts in a non-judgemental, non-reactive and accepting manner. Additionally, the course provides training in formal mindfulness practices, including body scan, sitting meditation and yoga. The principal objective of this meditation practice is to change the participant's relationship to stressful thoughts and events by decreasing emotional reactivity and enhancing cognitive appraisal.

Basic technique

Although it is recommended that you find an expert in your area, you can try this at home to get a sense of the experience.

Sit comfortably, close your eyes and focus your attention on your breathing. When we first focus on our breathing, we tend to become distracted by sensations and thoughts. Whenever this happens, simply redirect your focus to your breathing, without getting irritated or frustrated.

Proposed benefit

Mindfulness or open monitoring meditative practices cultivate a more present-centred awareness and bring you into the moment. One of the prevailing features of chronic stress is anticipatory worry about events that may, or may not, unfold in the future. In light of this, open monitoring practices offer an invaluable platform for resilience.

The conceptual model also suggests that the more you practise this, the easier it will be to cope with stressors because you're training your brain to avoid attachment to and judgement of sensations and thoughts.

Changes in brain function and behaviour

One of the most comprehensive reviews of the cognitive and behavioural influences of meditation on brain structure and function (95) confirms that open monitoring meditation practices increase activity and enhance key regions[42] in the brain. The effect of this neurological reorganisation includes enhanced movement potential, improved memory and learning, and better emotion formation and processing. Additionally, these brain regions positively influence compassion, empathy and perception – all exceedingly valuable in the management of chronic stress and enhanced resilience.

Integrative Body-Mind Training (IBMT)

According to an article in the journal *Neuroscience Bulletin* (96), IBMT is a practice based on traditional Chinese medicine in conjunction with the latest neuroscience research. It was originally developed as a methodology in the 1990s, and its effects have been extensively studied in Asia since 1995. The authority on IBMT is Professor Yi-Yuan Tang[43] of Texas Tech University.

According to Professor Yang:

> *IBMT avoids struggles to control thought, relying instead on a state of restful alertness that allows for a high degree of body-mind awareness while receiving instructions from a qualified coach, who provides body-adjustment guidance, mental imagery and other techniques while soothing music plays in the background. Thought control is achieved gradually through posture, relaxation, body-mind harmony and balance.*

The desired state is achieved by an initial 'mind setting', which encompasses a brief period of instructions to induce a cognitive or emotional set that will influence the practice.

IBMT practice emphasises that you distance your thoughts or emotions in order to come to the realisation that they are not you. In this way, your perspective is positively changed, providing for greater insight and clarity.

Proposed benefit

Since IBMT improves attention, cognitive performance and self-control, it could prove exceptionally valuable in the treatment of a range of stress-related psychopathologies.

Changes in brain function and behaviour

Seeing that IBMT is a form of open monitoring meditation, the neurological effects and benefits are expected to be much the same as those derived from mindfulness meditation.

Zen meditation

Zen meditation is a meditation practice that emphasises focused attention, which typically involves minimal distraction while observing the breath.

There are, however, different types of Zen meditation, each with its own unique focus. Fundamentally, the collective emphasis is on concentration, introspection, or even just sitting quietly.

Basic technique

As with any meditation practice, you should consult an expert or group in your area. However, to get a basic sense of this meditation experience, you can try this at home:

Sit cross-legged on a mat, cushion or chair. Traditionally, the practice involves sitting in a lotus or half-lotus position, but most of us would need to modify this position somewhat for comfort. Be sure to maintain a relaxed, upright posture. Make a point of not getting too comfortable, as it may be difficult to stay awake. Ideally, breathe with your abdominal muscles rather than your chest. Keep your mouth closed and your gaze on the ground about a metre in front of you. There are several ways in which to perform this type of meditation, which include focused attention and observation practices. I am going to provide only a brief description of a focus-based session.

For a focus-based meditation session, direct your attention to your breath as it flows in and out through your nose. Counting each full breath can make the meditation a lot easier for beginners. Use a total count of ten – five seconds in and five seconds out. While counting assists with focus, there will be moments when your attention drifts. Simply bring your attention back to your breath each time this happens.

Proposed benefit

According to an article published in the journal *Trends in Cognitive Sciences* (97), this type of focused attention meditation may lead to improvements in three areas: attention, disengaging from distraction, and shifting attention back to its intended target.

Changes in brain function and behaviour

Focused attention meditation practices promote enhanced functionality in regions of the brain that are associated with the regulation of thought and action. The areas showing the most significant increases in activity (46) are those involved in complex cognitive behaviour, decision-making, planning, social behaviour and even movement potential.[44] What is particularly interesting is the impact of focused attention meditation on a region of the brain known as the anterior cingulate cortex. This area of the brain contributes to the detection of conflict and responding to and managing emotional reactions – valuable attributes during periods of chronic stress.

Moreover, a research team from the University of Nevada (98) discovered that the functional role of this region of the brain is to create expectations and predictions about what's going to happen in the future based on past and current experiences. This may be particularly helpful in managing chronic stress, which is governed by emotional dysregulation and irrationality.

Loving kindness meditation

Loving kindness is a popular form of meditation. The aim is to deepen feelings of sympathetic joy for all living beings, as well as promote altruistic behaviours. Typically, novice practitioners begin by generating feelings of kindness, love and joy towards themselves, then progressively extending those feelings to visualised loved ones, acquaintances, strangers and, eventually, all living beings.

Basic technique

Should you wish to try this style of meditation at home, begin by sitting in a comfortable position with your eyes closed. Use your mind to create feelings of unconditional kindness and goodwill towards yourself. This can be achieved by mentally repeating phrases such as: "May I be happy." "May I be healthy." "May I be safe." "May I experience my full potential."

For most, it will take a bit of time to be able to send and receive feelings of kindness and care towards yourself. For some, it may be a highly charged emotional experience that can be somewhat overwhelming.

Once you have become adept at directing feelings of loving kindness towards yourself, visualise your spouse, child, a family member, or a good friend and direct feelings of unconditional kindness and goodwill to them as well.

The next stage involves directing these feelings towards a neutral person, possibly a stranger or an acquaintance. As you develop in this practice, you will eventually be able to send simultaneous feelings of loving kindness towards everyone including yourself, a close friend, a neutral person, a difficult person, and beyond. The ultimate goal is to wish genuine goodwill, peace and happiness towards all.

Proposed benefit

Mounting evidence from behavioural studies suggests that this meditative practice can be effective in developing empathy for others and, most notably, promoting pro-social behaviour. Remarkably, even brief training in compassion-based practices can inspire substantial changes in our behaviour. One of the first studies to provide confirmation about this was published in 2011 (99).

According to the team of researchers from the University of Zurich:

Our results provide first evidence for the positive impact of short-term compassion training on pro-social behaviour towards strangers in a training-unrelated task.

Simply put, a few minutes a day, or a session or two a week, can change our relationships with ourselves and others in a way that buffers us from stress, largely driven through the oxytocin system, increased vagal tone and reorganisation[45] in the brain itself.

Changes in brain function and behaviour

Neuro-imaging studies (95) show that loving kindness and compassion-based meditation practices impact three specific regions of the brain, including the regions that enhance emotional intelligence and all sensory information, and affect language and even mathematical capabilities.

Music

Few activities can transform our emotional state to the extent that music can. In an instant, music can make us feel relaxed, exhilarated, sad, happy, motivated, and every emotion in between. Music is frequently used by athletes, professionals and scholars to promote attention and focus, as well as relaxation. Not only does music have the potential to alter our mood and mental aptitudes, but also our physical abilities.

Often on the way to practice or training with a group of athletes, I hear the call to turn the car around – "I've forgotten my earphones!" My wife won't exercise without music. The question is: Does it really make such a difference? According to the literature it does, and the choice of music plays a significant role!

Synchronisation

In 2012, Australian researchers published a study in the *Journal of Science and Medicine in Sport* (100) on the effects of music on running potential. The study involved eleven elite triathletes who ran to exhaustion while being exposed to different musical environments. These included motivational music (fast-tempo, 120 bpm), neutral music (slower tempo and no catchy lyrics) and a no-music control.

The research team measured a host of variables, which included the time it took to reach exhaustion, mood responses, perceived rate of exertion,[46] running economy, and key performance markers like lactic acid concentrations in the blood, and oxygen use.

Incredibly, when compared to the no-music environment, the motivational music experience increased the time to exhaustion by an astounding 18.1%. The most notable biological shift was the effect that motivational music had on blood lactate levels, which were substantially reduced, suggesting improved energy efficiency. That said, it isn't completely unexpected since most of us have experienced how a training session is enhanced by enjoyable, high-energy music.

However, what did come as a surprise was the fact that the neutral music caused an even greater improvement in physical performance. According to the study, the neutral music increased the time to exhaustion to 19.7%. What the researchers found was that neutral music reduced the rate of perceived exertion and enhanced running economy.

Irrespective of the type of music, this performance advantage is something that scientists have been trying to understand for several years now. According to a research paper entitled "Anchoring: moving from theory to therapy" (101), music creates a sensory-movement synchronisation. In essence, although running and music have independent rhythms, when combined their rhythms will invariably sync to share a common frequency. This is because runners adjust their stride rate to the tempo of the music. This process is modulated by a specific region of the brain known as the supplementary motor area, which plays a central role in the perception of musical rhythm and the ordering of movements.

While this may not appear relevant in the stress resilience space, such findings give us an idea of the scale of music's influence on human biological systems. As far as I know, no performance enhancer can provide a 19% improvement in physical performance without any harmful side effects. Yet music's greatest value actually lies in the emotional and cognitive spaces.

Music and stress

Research into how music affects stress management is gaining tremendous traction, specifically in the areas of pain management, recovery, relaxation, psychotherapy and stress axis modulation.

To say that the influence of music on human health is multifactorial and complex is an understatement. A review article by researchers at McGill University in Canada (102) identifies four distinct ways in which music impacts our health. Music:

- improves motivation and pleasure
- promotes changes in levels of arousal by interacting with the stress axis
- influences the functionality and behaviour of our immune system, and
- impacts social and interpersonal relationships.

BY THE TIME FRIDAY COMES around, I'm generally feeling the effects of a busy week. My work schedule in South Africa typically starts on Sunday and involves treating patients, consulting to companies, public speaking, radio and TV, extensive travel and writing the odd article. As a general rule, whatever reserves I have in my energy tank, I take full advantage of, leaving me a little flat and somewhat fatigued. As I get to my consulting room, I select a favourite classical piece and hit play. Within minutes, I shift from lethargic to motivated; from tired and drained to clear and focused. Not only do the effects impact the way I feel, they also improve my dynamic with patients and the effectiveness of my diagnoses and treatments.

Music's effect on the brain

From a biological standpoint, music has a profound effect on several brain chemicals and hormones. These include dopamine and opioids[47] (including beta-endorphins), cortisol, serotonin, as well as the powerful stress resilience hormone, oxytocin.

When we consider the significant biological influence that music has on brain chemistry, it makes sense that the average person spends a great deal of time listening to music, regarding the experience as one of life's most enjoyable activities.

Over the years, scientists have gained a better understanding of the anatomical and chemical changes that occur in the brain in response to pleasurable music. Several studies using nuclear medicine functional imaging[48] have shown that there is a significant increase in regional blood flow and activity in several influential areas of the brain (102) whether you listen to your choice of music, unfamiliar pleasurable music, or even just burst into song yourself.

These increases in blood flow occur in regions that control, amongst other things:

- emotional and cognitive processing[49]
- movement
- visual and sound processing (mid-brain)
- sleep and alertness (thalamus), and
- posture, balance and coordination (cerebellum).

Functional Magnetic Resonance Imaging (fMRI) studies have also identified significant functional relationships between music and brain activity. One of the first to clearly define this connection was published in *NeuroImage* in 2005 (103). The research team from Stanford University showed that listening to music strongly influences dopamine release and heightened activity in several regions of the brain that are responsible for making us feel good about ourselves and our immediate circumstances.

Music, stress and vagal tone
The effects of music on stress have been extensively studied in an attempt to find sustainable solutions to the current global stress crisis. Knowledge and

understanding in this space are still evolving with new papers being published all the time.

In 2014, the *International Journal of Clinical and Experimental Physiology* (104) published a research study on the effects of music on stress in a group of medical students. Eighty medical students were divided into two groups: one group received daily exposure to classical music and the second group was a non-music control group. The music group were instructed to listen to preselected classical music pieces for 30 minutes every day for a month.

Vagus nerve integrity (which we now know is one of the primary markers of biological balance), as well as other tangible markers of stress (real or perceived) were monitored throughout the trial. Medical students are particularly suited to this type of experiment as they have limited authority over their own decisions, are always under significant time pressure, are constantly run down and fatigued, and are expected to perform at a high level mentally and physically day in and day out.

Over the month of the study, the music group showed lower overall heart rate and blood pressure values. They also presented with biological changes that characterise a lower state of overall arousal with greater vagal activity and potency.

Not only were there significant biological changes, the music group also reported a substantial (>20%) reduction in perceived stress.

Seeing that vagal tone is the cornerstone of stress resilience, these findings are extremely valuable in a stress resilience programme. Although this study used classical music, the trend in the literature is showing that any slow-tempo, enjoyable music will have similar effects.

Music boosts oxytocin following a stressful event
Not only is vagal tone enhanced through exposure to enjoyable music, it also

appears that oxytocin levels are also profoundly influenced by music.

Ulrica Nilsson, Assistant Professor at the Centre for Health Care Sciences in Orebro, Sweden, recently headed up a study that evaluated the effect of music on the recovery process in patients who had undergone major heart surgery (105).

The study was a randomised control trial involving 40 patients. Following open coronary artery bypass grafting and/or aortic valve replacement surgery, half the group were allocated to relaxing music exposure. The control group were not exposed to music. The focus of the trial was to evaluate regenerative potential and key relaxation markers. Circulating oxytocin, heart rate, blood pressure, arterial oxygen concentrations and subjective relaxation levels were also measured.

The researchers found that immediately after surgery levels of oxytocin plummeted within 30–60 minutes in the control group. By contrast, the music group showed the opposite effect – oxytocin levels spiked! This spike in oxytocin in response to listening to music was accompanied by higher levels of oxygen saturation in the bloodstream, as well as improved subjective relaxation.

According to the author:

> *Music intervention should be offered as an integral part of the multimodal regime administered to the patients that have undergone cardiovascular surgery. It is a supportive source that increases relaxation.*

These findings are groundbreaking! We now know that oxytocin offers tremendous stress-buffering effects on emotions and behaviour. We also know that it provides enormous physical support.

The effects of music on cortisol

Seeing that cortisol is one of the most effective biomarkers of chronic stress, it makes sense that there have been numerous research papers evaluating the effects of either listening to music or making music on cortisol levels. At least 29 high-quality studies have been identified (106) in which there is general consensus that regular exposure to relaxing music lowers cortisol!

Not all music has the same effect, though. Patient-selected music resulted in greater reductions in cortisol compared with experimenter-selected music. There is also evidence that high-tempo, stimulating music results in increased activity of the stress axis and elevated cortisol.

Several years ago, Italian researchers investigated the emotional and hormonal changes that occur in response to listening to techno[50] music (107). The small group of participants were randomly assigned to listen to either techno music or classical music for a period of 30 minutes. It should come as no surprise that the techno music group showed a rise in heart rate, blood pressure, beta-endorphins, adrenocorticotropic hormone, noradrenalin and cortisol compared with the classical music group. While this may be an advantageous state to be in when engaging in vigorous exercise or staying up all night, it certainly is not the kind of state you would want to induce during periods of chronic stress!

The immediate effects of music

So far we've established that music after a stressful event and/or daily listening to calming music impacts key stress moderators, such as vagal tone and oxytocin.

The big question is: to what extent does listening to music impact our ability to cope and deal with impending stresses? While arousal is a prerequisite for performance, success and adaptability, excessive arousal can have the opposite effect. A crucial concern in ongoing stress is the fact that the stress axis can become dysfunctional, lending itself to disproportionate responses to stimuli with correspondingly high levels of cortisol and adrenalin.

FOR ALMOST TWO DECADES I have sat in locker rooms next to elite athletes from a variety of sports disciplines prior to competition. You might think that there would be a lot of talk and motivational speeches, but in my experience the pre-game/match environment is nothing like that.

In many instances, there is hardly any conversation or engagement between the athletes or with the outside world. Instead, they prefer to enter their chosen 'safe-space' using a headset and a careful selection of motivational music.

Tennis is particularly renowned for this practice, and it is common to see players stepping onto the court with the latest headset wrapped around their neck or on their ears. One of the tennis players known for incorporating music into his pre-match routine is the iconic Rafael Nadal.

From my days working in professional tennis, one of the standout memories was seeing Rafa putting on his trendy headset and slowly getting into his zone before each and every match. I always wondered whether he listened to calming music or up-tempo stimulating playlists. I certainly wasn't going to ask him during his pre-match preparation!

Numerous studies have shown that listening to relaxing music prior to or during stressful medical procedures, and in controlled laboratory environments, results in a decrease in the stress response across the primary measurable parameters, including lower cortisol and adrenalin. This being said, there are also studies showing limited effects of music exposure prior to stressful events, which has created confusion among health professionals and scientists. However, it is believed that many of these discrepancies are due to methodological issues[51] with the studies themselves.

In 2013, a team of multinational researchers published a study (108) that demystified the science surrounding the contentious topic of whether listening to music prior to a stressful event reduces the stress response.

The study involved 60 healthy female volunteers with an average age of 25. The participants were randomly assigned to one of three environments:

- relaxing music
- rippling water (natural sound, no rhythmic or melodic structure), and
- no music.

The participants were then exposed to a standardised psychosocial stress test.

The research team evaluated a wide range of stress markers in all subjects. This included salivary cortisol and salivary alpha-amylase,[52] heart rate, vagus nerve integrity,[53] subjective stress perception and anxiety.

Remarkably, the research team was able to clearly identify the biological effects of various types of music and natural sounds on the stress axis. Oddly enough, the findings were not at all what the scientists anticipated.

Stress hormone responses

In terms of hormonal responses, the researchers found significant differences among the groups, specifically in cortisol levels. The team had expected cortisol levels to be lowest in the music group and highest in the no music group. However, this was not the case. The relaxing music group displayed the largest spike in cortisol in response to a stress simulation. The no music control showed a smaller spike in cortisol. Intriguingly, cortisol levels were lowest in the rippling water group, which follows no rhythmic or melodic structure.

Effects on the nervous system

When investigating the effects of the three acoustic environments on nervous system responses, the picture was somewhat different. Although the differences among the groups were not overt, the music group showed a trend to faster recovery from a stressor and greater vagal activity.

Psychological effects

Finally, when it came to the psychological measurements, such as perception of stress, there were no significant differences among the three groups.

What we can draw from this research is that listening to relaxing music prior to a stressful event may increase alertness and arousal, but will definitely promote a more rapid recovery and improved balance after the event. It is interesting that natural sounds may offer the best results when you want to lower the overall stress response and your level of arousal before a challenging task.

Music and sleep

It is widely accepted that stress is highly disruptive in the context of sleep. Stress and associated anxiety can induce a state of hyper-arousal, which can make it challenging to fall asleep, stay asleep, and can even impact the quality of sleep.

According to a 2017 report by the American Psychological Association (21a), 48% of persons who suffer from some form of insomnia attribute it directly to stress.

We can all recall a period where we have gone to bed at night after a stressful day with our minds racing and hearts pounding. Minutes of tossing and turning become hours. The frustration builds, knowing that the more agitated we become, the lower the likelihood of actually falling asleep.

If this happens once in a while, it is not overly impactful. However, if this becomes a trend, it can dramatically impair functioning and health.

Chronic stress and anxiety can profoundly impact sleep for extended periods, leaving you with little choice but to resort to sedatives – pharmaceutical or botanical. But this comes at a cost. In the short term, it may impact mental acuity and energy levels the following day. In the long term, the side effects may be extremely detrimental to health.

Sleep deprivation or disruptions – even for a few days – in otherwise healthy individuals can result in further wear and tear[54] on body systems. According to a research paper entitled "Sleep deprivation and circadian disruption: stress, allostasis, and allostatic load" (109), compromised sleep results in increased sympathetic tone,[55] increased pro-inflammatory proteins,[56] elevated evening cortisol, as well as increased blood sugar and insulin.

According to Dr Bruce McEwen, who headed up the study, when sleep is disrupted for protracted periods of time, the biological disturbances include:

- elevations in cortisol
- increased free-radical production
- impaired brain integrity (structure and function), and
- metabolic disorders, such as obesity.

The mounting evidence suggests that listening to calming music before bed may help considerably with all facets of sleep. In 2016, Chinese researchers published a study (110) on the effects of music intervention on overall sleep quality. The study was a randomised, controlled trial over a three-month period that involved 64 participants with sleep disorders. The sleep disorders were quantified by a rating of greater than 7 on the Pittsburgh Sleep Quality Index[57] (PSQI).

The participants were divided equally into a music group and a control group. All participants received one sleep hygiene session of 15 minutes that included education about preparing a comfortable environment for sleep; avoiding smoking, alcohol, tea, coffee, caffeinated beverages, being too full or too hungry before sleep; and the importance of maintaining regular sleep schedules. The participants also received bi-weekly telephone calls.

The music-intervention group were required to listen to music for 30–45 minutes each night. The music playlist was carefully selected and included soft, sedative pieces with stable melodies at a tempo of 60–80 bpm.[58]

While both groups benefited from the sleep hygiene education, the music-intervention group showed marked improvements in sleep quality. These improvements were ongoing, with each month's improvement surpassing the previous month. By the end of the study, 50% of the participants in the music group achieved normal sleep quality, with a PSQI global score of 7 or less.

This study differed from previous interventions because it evaluated sleep in all its component parts, which included:

- sleep latency – length of time from full wakefulness to sleep
- sleep efficiency – proportion of sleep time during time spent in bed, and
- daytime dysfunction – subjective perception of daytime activities after sleep.

Improvements were seen across all domains. Although this was a high-quality study and the conclusions are very clear, it is still necessary to look at the collective literature over a protracted period of time in order to gain the greatest degree of objectivity on any health intervention. The use of music as a tool to manage sleep disorders is no different.

Fortunately, with insomnia fast becoming a major global issue there are numerous published papers on this positive relationship. In 2017, Chinese researchers from several medical research centres and universities performed an extensive meta-analysis of the literature pertaining specifically to music and sleep disorder management (111). The researchers aimed to compare and rank music interventions for primary insomnia patients.

The review identified 20 trials involving a total of 1 339 patients, which incorporated a variety of sleep interventions. Listening to music, music combined with exercise, music-guided relaxation, conventional medication, acupuncture, and other medical approaches were all compared. Using PSQI scores as a primary measure, the research showed that regardless of the type of intervention, when music was included the outcomes were considerably better. The study also revealed that music-guided relaxation resulted in better overall sleep quality[59] compared with medication. Simply put: music-guided relaxation is a better insomnia management tool than strong medications.

Regarding sleep latency, listening to music and music-assisted relaxation are the most effective interventions in the review. Lastly, if you're looking to improve sleep efficiency, music combined with exercise offers the greatest returns.

The conclusions of the study clearly showed the advantages of musical interventions for those who struggle with insomnia. So much so that the authors suggest that music should be a first-line intervention for sleep disorders.

I HAVE EXPERIENCED THE BENEFITS of relaxing music for sleep several times in past months. I have to admit that it hasn't necessarily been through conscious intention on my part, but rather as an indirect consequence of trying to put Isaac, our young son, to sleep. As a general preference, Isaac prefers the night-time hours to play, eat and have fun with my wife and me.

Naturally, we would love to indulge him, but daytime responsibilities take precedence, however cute he may be. In our search for sleeping tools and strategies, we have discovered a repertoire of baby music playlists and, in doing so, have found a way to curb the night-time parties in Isaac's room. But there's a new sleep problem now – when we put on *his* playlist, all of us are sound asleep in a few minutes.

Isaac's playlist has become so valuable to us that when we don't have access to the iPad, we know we are in for an action-packed evening. Moreover, in recent months when I have gone through challenging sleeping periods, I resort to some of his favourite play-lists. The only downside is that some of the children's tunes get stuck in my head for the better part of the next day!

Music and brain waves

One stand-out feature of slow, soothing music is the positive effect it has on our brain waves. This is especially relevant during periods of chronic stress when excess beta[60] waves may prevail due to excess adrenalin. Meditation, aerobic exercise and certain dietary behaviours can induce predominantly alpha brain-wave frequencies, which are known for their ability to calm the body and promote relaxation.

Studies show that slow, soothing music can also alter regional brain-wave states not only by transporting the listener into the alpha wave frequency – as a recent study by Italian researchers shows (112) – but also into a theta state (113).

Theta waves are typically connected to sleep and deep emotional states. The theta frequency range promotes creativity and emotional connectivity, enhances intuition and induces a state of deep relaxation.

So if you're writing an exam or giving a keynote address, theta is really *not* the state you want to be in. However, if you're chronically over-aroused, stressed and anxious, being able to rapidly transition into alpha and theta brain wave frequencies – especially towards the end of the day – can be highly advantageous.

Music, the immune system and inflammation

Listening to music both reduces stress and improves mood, which should then create improved immune functionality.

Before I discuss the role of music in immune functionality, I have to briefly discuss how certain components of our immune system work. The large surface areas of the digestive, respiratory and urogenital systems represent major sites of potential attack by invading microorganisms.[61] Our first line of defence is a powerful antibody[62] known as immunoglobulin A (IgA). IgA is present in many of our external excretions and saturates our mucosal surfaces[63] providing valuable protection where we need it most.

Stress has an extremely disruptive effect on IgA balance. While acute stress increases secretions, offering considerable protection and strong immunity (114), chronic stress and even periods following acute stress are associated with a collapse in this all-important antibody. Numerous studies (115, 116) have investigated immune behaviours in professions where chronic stress is common. The consensus is that professionals who are exposed to a greater degree of chronic stress have lower IgA production predisposing them to viral and bacterial infections on an ongoing basis. This is part of the reason we often get sick following periods of acute stress or during periods of chronic stress.

According to a 2013 review by English researchers (106) of the literature on the effects of music on our emotions, and nervous and immune systems, there have been at least eight high-quality studies that report an increase in IgA levels following music exposure from a variety of different genres. What was interesting about these findings is that IgA levels were greatest when the participants enjoyed the music most. Moreover, if the participants were actively involved in making the music, this too created a large increase in IgA.

What is fascinating about music and immunity is the influence that listening to music has on allergic responses to food. A study published in *Inflammation Research* (117) investigated this relationship only to find that histamine release is reduced when exposed to allergenic foods in combination with music. Other studies support these or similar findings. Does this mean that the next time you eat foods that you know don't agree with your system, all you have to do is blast Mozart? Not quite – but it does highlight the powerful relationship between music and the immune system.

Chronic stress is often associated with chronic inflammation. At the centre of chronic inflammation and its associated inflammatory diseases is an immune-mediated protein called interleukin-6 (IL-6). While this important protein is essential as a defence against infection or injury in the short term, if dysregulated due to biological changes[64] that occur through chronic stress, this molecule can have a profoundly negative effect on health. In fact, according to an article in *Arthritis Research & Therapy* (118), levels of circulating IL-6 are significantly elevated in several inflammatory diseases, including rheumatoid arthritis, systemic juvenile arthritis, systemic lupus erythematosus, ankylosing spondylitis, psoriasis and Crohn's disease. Moreover, in autoimmune diseases, IL-6 not only maintains the state of inflammation, but also further corrupts and changes overall immune responses within the body.

A vicious cycle ensues: Chronic stress elevates levels of circulating IL-6, which then triggers the stress axis ... and the cycle is perpetuated.

With this pro-inflammatory protein driving ill health and biological strain, any and all interventions that have the capacity to reduce IL-6 should form the basis of a stress resilience programme.

In 2009, researchers from the Department of Internal Medicine and Cardiology at Nippon Medical School in Japan published a study (119) investigating the effects of music therapy on 87 patients with cardiovascular disease. The participants were randomly assigned to two groups – a music therapy[65] group and a non-therapy group. The music therapy group received at least one 45-minute music therapy session a week for ten sessions. As you would expect, the non-music therapy group experienced little to no change during the period of the study, but the music therapy group experienced significant change across many domains. Increases in vagal tone and overall decreases in adrenalin were observed. Not only were these two important stress resilience changes noted, there was also a marked reduction in IL-6, indicating lower levels of systemic inflammation. It is no wonder that the music therapy group experienced a lower rate of congestive heart failure during the study.

It appears that listening to classical music has the same effect, particularly in critically ill persons. A research paper entitled "Overture for growth hormone: requiem for interleukin-6" (120) found that listening to Mozart

– specifically some of his slower works – had a profound impact on key health markers.

The study involved a small group of critically ill patients who were randomly assigned to a music group or non-music group a day after surgery. The music group listened to one hour of Mozart that had been carefully selected based on its structure and known influence on relaxation. The research team measured circulatory variables, brain electrical activity, levels of stress hormones and cytokines (inflammatory proteins), requirements for sedative drugs, and level of sedation before and after the one-hour music session.

The results were nothing short of incredible! When the music group was compared with the control group their blood pressure and heart rate were lower due to higher vagal tone, and adrenalin had decreased. This said, what was most striking was the fact that growth hormone[66] levels spiked and IL-6 decreased significantly. This study further shows the degree of influence that music has within the context of stress resilience and health promotion.

Practical application

- To increase vagal activity, listen to enjoyable, slow-tempo (60–80 bpm), melodic music for at least 30 minutes a day.
- If you have a stressful event like public speaking or an exam, try listening to relaxing music for 10 minutes before the event. This will increase arousal and alertness for the impending task and will speed up the recovery process following the stress experience.
- If you want to reduce cortisol and lower the activity of the stress axis during an event, listen to nature sounds for 10 minutes or longer prior to the upcoming challenge.
- If you want to improve sleep quality, listen to relaxing, enjoyable music 30–45 minutes before sleep. The music must be melodic with tempos of 60–80 bpm. Classical and instrumental are recommended.
- Listening to Mozart's slower pieces for an hour will lower systemic

inflammation and increase growth hormone output. The same effect can be achieved with music therapy. For more on music therapy, go to https://www.musictherapy.org.

- Listening to fast tempo (120 bpm) enjoyable music, as well as neutral music during exercise dramatically enhances performance.
- Actively singing promotes a considerably greater reduction of stress hormones than listening does.
- Active participation in the making of music has a marked influence on IgA levels, to such an extent that if you suffer from ongoing colds and flu, it may be worthwhile learning to play a musical instrument.

Genes, inflammation and lifestyle choices

Although mind-body interventions offer tremendous health benefits from a genetic perspective, we also have to consider the robust influence of lifestyle practices, such as diet and exercise. These are discussed in *Chapter 8 Step 4: Rebuild and Repair.*

In a recent study, Canadian researchers from Laval University in Quebec found that diets high in processed sugar and refined carbohydrates, saturated fat and meats are associated with significant genetic shifts favouring chronic inflammation and disease (121). The same study found the opposite to be the case in diets high in fruits, vegetables, whole grains and fish.[67]

The saturated fats found in red meat and other animal products appear to be particularly influential in initiating abnormal genetic behaviours. Over the last decade, several studies have reported a strong association between animal fat intake and increased levels of inflammation. A 2009 Dutch study investigated the biological effects of diets high in saturated fats,[68] comparing them with diets rich in mono-unsaturated fats[69] (122).

Although the study measured a variety of health markers, such as insulin sensitivity and blood lipids, the emphasis was on gene expression profiles. The trial was small, involving only 20 participants between the ages of 45 and

60 who were overweight and at risk of developing metabolic syndrome.

Metabolic syndrome is typically characterised by obesity, insulin resistance, elevated blood lipids and high blood pressure. It is a major factor in the development of cardiovascular diseases and diabetes.

The study design required that all subjects consume a diet high in saturated fat[70] for two weeks. The subjects were then allocated to one of the intervention diets, which they sustained for a period of eight weeks.

Ten subjects were put on the high saturated-fat diet, which was similar to the two-week preliminary diet. The other ten subjects were placed on a mono-unsaturated fat diet high in olive oil. In order to provide accurate results, both diets were comparable in terms of overall macronutrients, such as carbohydrates, protein, total fat and dietary fibre.

What the Dutch research team discovered was that participants on the high saturated-fat diet[71] showed a robust increase in the expression of many genes involved in inflammation processes. By contrast, the mono-unsaturated fat diet resulted in a higher anti-inflammatory gene expression profile, which was also accompanied by a decrease in LDL-cholesterol[72] levels.

The effects of various forms of exercise on genetic behaviours are also significant. An extensive meta-analysis by Norwegian researchers (123) showed that there are significant alterations in genetic expression following activity. The genes with increased activity following exercise are typically involved in inflammation, cell communication, cell protection, growth and repair.

Interestingly, the majority of the 37 studies show that a single bout of exercise induces an immediate pro-inflammatory response. However, this effect is short-lived as prolonged and regular physical activity actually promotes a genetically mediated anti-inflammatory environment. The positive genetic behaviours seen in response to regular physical exercise appear to be similar to those of mind-body interventions.

For this reason, researchers are unsure whether or not the anti-inflammatory effects of the activity-based mind-body interventions, such as yoga and tai chi, are due to the physical component or the meditative effects.

CHAPTER SUMMARY

- One of the fundamental building blocks in the promotion of stress resilience is the integrity of the vagus nerve. The higher its tone and functionality, the greater our ability to restore and maintain a state of biological balance. The vagus nerve also promotes synchronicity between the body and the brain. However, one of its best-recognised attributes is its ability to calm the body after the fight-or-flight state induced by the stress hormone adrenalin. Robust vagus nerve activity dramatically lowers cortisol and inflammation.
- Various practices can be used to increase vagal activation and tone during stressful periods, which will build overall stress resilience.
- Because there are numerous practices that increase vagal activation and tone, this book covers the following modalities as a representative sample to form the basis of an effective stress management programme:
  - visceral manipulation
  - massage therapy
  - controlled breathing exercises
  - swimming
  - facial immersion
  - yoga
  - meditation
  - music.
- **Visceral manipulation** practitioners have a skill set to stimulate the vagus nerve directly, mobilise organs and glands, manipulate the spinal column, release intrinsic muscular tension and manually desensitise the sympathetic nervous system to correct the stress response.
- **Massage therapy** is an effective stress management/resilience tool. Not only does massage therapy increase vagus nerve activity and raise

oxytocin, but it also significantly lowers cortisol. Moreover, massage promotes an increase in serotonin and dopamine, which positively influence cognition and behaviour.

- **Controlled breathing** exercises increase vagal tone and parasympathetic activity, leading to a dramatic reduction in adrenalin and cortisol levels.
  - Controlled breathing exercises may be effective in managing high blood pressure and related health issues
  - Research shows controlled breathing exercises to be effective in managing depression and anxiety disorders
  - Deep diaphragmatic breathing can create improved engagement of numerous regions of the brain, including those responsible for memory and emotional processes.
- **Swimming** activates the vagus nerve and reduces activity of the stress axis through a survival response called the 'dive reflex'. Additional benefits are achieved through exercise and rhythmic breathing in the water.
  - Regular swimming has been shown to dramatically reduce the risk of chronic diseases as well as improve life expectancy.
- **Cold water** (10°C/50°F) or pack (1–2°C/34°–36°F) facial immersion for a period of 30 seconds to 3 minutes triggers vagus nerve activity through its relationship with the trigeminal nerve. This nerve has been used as a reliable measure of vagus nerve functionality and provides a quick and easy solution to managing stressful situations.
- **Regular yoga practice is successful in managing chronic stress and promoting stress resilience.**
- Yoga is more than a simple exercise routine. It encompasses:
  - physical postures and exercises
  - breathing exercises
  - deep relaxation techniques, and
  - meditation and/or mindfulness practices.

- These activities promote physical strength and flexibility, enhance respiratory functioning, increase the ability to release tension, and improve cognitive and emotional integrity.
- Yoga increases activity of the vagus nerve; regular practice increases vagal tone.
- Studies show that yoga is successful in improving behaviour and reducing stress in children.
- Studies have shown that yoga practice is effective in reducing the symptoms of depression and lowering cortisol in depressed patients.
- Daily yoga practice in healthy individuals can result in a 40% reduction in cortisol levels.
- **Meditation** is a form of mental training that aims to improve an individual's attention and emotional self-regulation.
  - Meditation has beneficial effects in a number of important cognitive domains, including attention, memory, verbal fluency, executive function, processing speed, overall cognitive flexibility and conflict monitoring, and can even enhance creativity.
  - Meditation can lower cortisol and reduce stress responses.
  - Meditation dramatically improves connectivity and functionality within the brain.
  - Meditation enhances the structural properties of the brain in no less than eight specific regions and protects the brain against ageing.
  - Meditation positively affects our DNA in such a way that it reduces inflammation and improves immune regulation.
  - Meditation practice in younger individuals increases brain size and volume.
  - Each form of meditation brings with it its own unique benefits, which can be tailored to your needs.
- **Music** is a powerful tool in promoting stress resilience.
- Listening to slow, calming music increases vagal tone and oxytocin levels.

- Relaxing music also lowers cortisol and increases dopamine, opioids, serotonin and beta-endorphins.
- Pleasurable music increases blood flow to areas of the brain responsible for:
  - emotional and cognitive processing
  - movement
  - posture and balance
  - visual and auditory processing, and
  - sleep.
- Listening to relaxing music prior to a stressful event increases alertness and arousal and enhances recovery after the event.
- Listening to nature sounds prior to a stressful event lowers cortisol and stress hormone responses.
- Listening to calming music:
  - can promote deep relaxation by altering brain wave states in favour of alpha, and possibly even theta, waves
  - increases IgA antibody levels providing increased protection against pathogens
  - reduces inflammation, specifically the pro-inflammatory molecule known as IL-6
  - before bed improves all aspects of sleep and is highly effective in managing insomnia.
  - Listening to classical music reduces allergic reactions to food.
  - Listening to Mozart has been shown to increase growth hormone levels.
  - Listening to music during aerobic exercise increases performance and time to exhaustion.

STEP 4:
REBUILD AND REPAIR

We've seen how periods of chronic stress are typically accompanied by a decline in physical vitality, emotional stability and cognitive integrity. Even when the stressor is removed, these states often persist and require active and focused intervention. Fortunately, restoration of vitality, health and cognitive potency can be achieved through numerous *sustained* lifestyle behaviours and practices. Random lifestyle changes, however constructive, might not effect the desired returns on any level.

The key to neutralising the long-term effects of stress lies in the creation of a molecular bias. This state needs to focus on the very hormones and molecules that become down-regulated by the two waves in the stress response – the SAM and HPA axes. These include brain-derived neurotrophic factor (BDNF) and other neurotrophins, growth hormone (somatotrophin), and the neurotransmitters serotonin and dopamine.

Many activities, nutritional supplements (nutraceuticals), dietary practices and even certain environmental conditions can increase the production and circulating levels of several of these molecules and hormones.

This chapter provides a variety of simple lifestyle practices that will enhance cognitive potential, emotional stability and physical integrity.

REBUILDING THE BRAIN AND BODY

Cortisol decimates brain integrity by causing structural changes and compositional alterations, as well as promoting large-scale atrophy. We need to do our utmost to reverse these ravaging effects on our most precious resource. Incredibly, the body produces a group of protein molecules, neurotrophins, which can fully reverse the damage brought on by chronic stress. Within this neurotrophin group,[1] the most active of these signalling proteins in terms of stimulating neurogenesis[2] is BDNF.

BDNF is a protein produced inside nerve cells that promotes the structural integrity and functionality of the brain through new brain cell formation, maturation and retention, as well as by building connections between the cells.

According to Dr John Ratey, an Associate Professor at Harvard Medical School (124), when nerve cells are placed in a petri dish and immersed in BDNF, they spontaneously sprout branches in the same way they would when learning a new skill or task. What's more, BDNF significantly increases the strength of electrical impulses passing between nerve cells[3] thereby creating greater functionality and connectivity. Finally, once inside the cell, BDNF activates genes that signal the production of more BDNF, as well as the powerful behavioural neurotransmitter serotonin.

Simply put, through a variety of mechanisms, BDNF is the basis for brain cell integrity and functionality, as well as cognitive and possibly even behavioural potential.

Elevating BDNF levels through exercise

Moderate-intensity aerobic exercise
While many nutritional and environmental factors are able to elevate BDNF,

exercise has the most powerful influence by far. Researchers at the University of California were able to demonstrate that both daily exercise and alternating days of aerobic exercise increased BDNF protein production. Additionally, the study (125) showed that BDNF levels progressively increased with longer durations of exercise. After three months of daily exercise, secretion rates at rest were dramatically elevated (222%). The same study also showed that after a month of regular, moderate-intensity aerobic exercise, BDNF levels remained elevated by as much as 133% for seven days, even without activity.

High-intensity aerobic exercise

High-intensity aerobic interval exercise appears to be far more effective at elevating BDNF than continuous aerobic exercise. While numerous studies show that moderate intensity aerobic exercise is associated with a substantial rise in BDNF levels (>30% in a single session), this release is significantly amplified with interval training. According to a recent collaborative study between Belgian and Swiss researchers (126), interval training is associated with a rise in BDNF levels of more than 60% within a 20-minute period.

Exercising in hot weather augments release of BDNF

According to a study published in *Neuroscience Letters* (127), exercising in hot weather further augments BDNF release. The study found that temperatures in the region of 30°C/86°F caused the greatest spike in BDNF.

Resistance training influences BDNF

Although aerobic training has been shown to be the greatest trigger in both short-term and long-term elevations of BDNF, resistance training has recently been shown to influence secretion rates as well. According to a 2016 study published in the *Journal of Applied Physiology* (128), increases in BDNF occur with weight training protocols irrespective of the level of intensity or volume of exercise.

There have been contradictions in the literature with studies reporting little to no change in BDNF levels. However, these findings are due to the differences in exercise selection. All the studies reporting no change in BDNF in response to resistance exercise involved isolated muscle contractions performed on machines. For example, a small Brazilian study (129) involving only sixteen participants found no appreciable changes in BDNF concentrations in the bloodstream in response to the prescribed exercise protocol. However, the protocol involved isolated muscle contractions for the thighs and arms on exercise machines. By contrast, studies (128) using multi-joint complex movements, such as squats, presses and deadlifts, showed dramatic increases in BDNF concentrations lasting for up to 60 minutes after the exercise.

Comparing aerobic and resistance exercise in BDNF output

In terms of their influence on BDNF blood levels, aerobic and resistance training display different secretion rates at rest. For example, according to a 2010 study published in the *American Journal of Physiology – Regulatory, Integrative and Comparative Physiology* (130), a fourfold increase in resting BDNF secretion was observed after three months of endurance training at moderate intensities (65% of VO2 max). Although resistance training provides robust short-term elevations, the long-term elevations produced by aerobic exercise cannot be replicated.

The harder you train the greater the gain

According to numerous studies, including a 2013 article published in the *Journal of Sports Science and Medicine* (131), aerobic exercise is typically associated with a 30% or greater rise in BDNF levels, peaking at around eighteen minutes. Additionally, the more vigorous the intensity – 80% of maximum heart rate – and/or the longer the duration (>40 min) the more significant the BDNF elevation. Examples of aerobic exercise include brisk walking, running, cycling, swimming, working out on an elliptical machine, circuit training and hiking.

Without question, aerobic interval training is the most effective means of elevating BDNF in the short term, with secretion rates rising by as much as 60%. Training examples include spinning, soccer, tennis, interval runs[4] and swimming at different speeds or with different strokes, as well as a host of other intense activities.

My exercise and activity recommendation is: incorporate both sustained and interval training into your weekly training routine, as both are associated with enhanced BDNF secretion rates.

Balancing intensity and burnout

Another advantage offered by interval training is that the BDNF peaks are more prolonged. However, a word of caution! Interval training is intense and very taxing on the body, so sessions require a prolonged warm-up, and low frequency (not too many sessions in a week) to avoid burnout or injury.

Use these guidelines to work out the best frequency for you:

- if you're not exercise-inclined, do only one session per week
- if you're a fitness enthusiast, do no more than two sessions per week, and
- if you're more athletically inclined, do no more than three sessions per week.

For those who live in hot climates, a session per week in which aerobic training is performed outdoors can offer a significant boost in BDNF secretion. Just make sure you are well hydrated and have appropriate sun protection.

Another important consideration is that daily training promotes greater and more rapid increases in overall secretion rates. The key to regular exercise is properly managed fluctuations in intensity and volume:

- on days when you have energy, you can perform the more vigorous sessions, and
- on the days you feel tired or run down, a mere twenty minutes

of walking will be enough to promote increases in BDNF levels and facilitate the positive trajectory towards brain integrity and functionality.

Here are some basic aerobic interval training examples:

Cycling

1. 10 minutes of easy warm-up (40–50% maximum heart rate)
2. 30 seconds of intense effort (80–100%) followed by 90 seconds of easy riding; repeat 6 to 10 times
3. 5 minutes of light cool-down
4. 10 minutes of stretches to support recovery

Running treadmill

1. 10 minutes of easy warm-up (40–50% maximum heart rate)
2. 1 minute of high effort (75–90%), followed by 1 minute of easy effort (40–50%); repeat 4 to 10 times
3. 5 minutes of light cool-down
4. 10 minutes of stretches to support recovery

Swimming

1. 10 minutes of warm-up (±500 metres, any stroke)
2. 100 metres of freestyle as fast as you can; rest for 1 to 2 minutes; repeat 4 to 10 times
3. 5 to 10 minutes of cool-down (any stroke)
4. 10 minutes of stretches to support recovery

Choosing the right weight training routine

Resistance training can be an effective means of increasing BDNF and promoting stress resilience. Although volume and intensity have equal influence with respect to secretion rates, the type of exercise selected is a major determinant in BDNF secretion. Choose complex, multi-point movements, preferably in a circuit fashion, to achieve the best results.

Elevating growth hormone levels through exercise

Numerous research articles have reliably shown an inverse relationship between high cortisol levels and lowered growth hormone (GH) secretion. In fact, scientists believe that the entire GH axis is controlled by daily fluctuations in cortisol (132). Seeing that GH is responsible for numerous biological functions, including cell reproduction and growth, DNA integrity, strong bones, youthful skin, neurological integrity, muscle tone, muscle size, and optimal functioning of the cardiovascular and immune systems, it is imperative that levels be restored after stressful periods.

Although deep sleep, certain nutraceuticals, and fasting are strong influences on GH secretion, one of the most potent stimulators of GH output is *exercise*. The type, intensity and duration all have a very specific influence on GH secretion, as well as the behavioural characteristics of this hormone once in circulation.

In a 2007 study published in the *European Journal of Applied Physiology* (133), researchers compared the GH response from aerobic exercise and resistance exercise sessions in the same subjects. A randomised aerobic group was assigned to perform either 30 minutes of continuous cycling at 70% of their maximal effort (VO2 max), and another group, the resistance training group, was assigned to perform free weight training at 70% of their maximal effort for one repetition (1RM). The next week, the groups performed the other training so that all subjects had completed both exercise protocols.

Blood samples measuring GH output in response to the different exercise practices were taken at various intervals. Samples were drawn prior to exercise, during exercise, and following the exercise sessions. After adjusting for the amount of work performed per minute of exercise, it was shown that both types of exercise caused a significant increase in GH output, peaking towards the end of the session and during the recovery period, at around 30 to 60 minutes. However, the results also showed that GH secretion was far greater and exhibited better bioactivity from the resistance training protocol.

Exercise-induced GH secretion typically begins 10 to 20 minutes after exercise onset, with peak concentrations occurring immediately post-exercise or shortly thereafter. According to a review article in *Sports Medicine* (134), the literature shows a linear dose response between exercise intensity and GH secretion. This means that the harder you train, the greater the GH spike in response to exercise, much the same as BDNF. The same article also highlights that an optimal exercise stimulus significantly increases GH concentrations within the circulatory system in all age groups, even those who are experiencing age-related GH reductions, as is common in older men.

Not all training protocols, however intense, evoke the same responses. Resistance training and machine exercise sessions that isolate smaller muscles, have long rest periods and work with light or, conversely, extremely heavy loads, will do very little to change the GH axis and produce an enhanced physical state. Yet, for many years, this has been the most common training methodology and practice within the health and fitness sector. Instead, resistance exercise protocols that stimulate large muscle groups (involving expansive movements), use moderate loads (a maximum of ten repetitions), and have relatively short rest periods (less than a minute), together with a high amount of total work have been shown to maximise the GH response to exercise.

Here is an example:

1. 10 push-ups (feet up on a bench)
2. 10 squats
3. 10 body weight dips or pull-ups
4. 10 walking lunges
5. Rest for 1 minute
6. Repeat several times before moving on to another circuit of a similar nature.

When wanting to increase secretion rates through aerobic exercise, moderation may not be the most effective approach. Both high intensity and higher overall training volume independently appear to evoke the greatest GH responses.

Several years ago, researchers at the UCLA School of Medicine published a study on aerobic exercise and corresponding hormonal adaptations (135). The researchers discovered that when comparing different aerobic protocols, only the sessions that involved 10 minutes or longer above the lactate threshold (±75% of maximum heart rate) resulted in a substantial increase in circulating GH levels. What was remarkable about this study was the volume of exercise-induced growth hormone secretion, which was approximately 700% higher than the baseline levels. In this study, neither the shorter sessions (<10 minutes) nor the moderate-intensity training sessions for durations exceeding 10 minutes could replicate this positive biological response.

This is not the only means by which aerobic exercise can result in large GH surges. There are two other ways, vastly different in nature, yet similar in effect.

A randomised, controlled trial comparing different durations of exercise and varied protocols was recently published in *Medicine and Science in Sports and Exercise* (136). Although the study was small, it was rigorously controlled in terms of diet, sleep and exercise practices. The 20-hour evaluation compared moderate intensity and duration training protocols (both resistance and aerobic) to longer duration (in excess of 2 hours) protocols. The study also included a control group. The findings revealed that only the long duration aerobic exercise resulted in a significant amplification of GH secretion in a variety of domains, including peaks, total 20-hour secretion rates, and so on. The researchers speculate that this rise in 20-hour GH levels is related to energy expenditure, suggesting that higher energy protocols may create elevated growth hormone profiles. However, more research needs to be done before any firm conclusions can be drawn.

If you don't want to go for a two-hour run, swim or cycle, the good news is that there is another way to elevate GH through aerobic exercise in a fraction of the time – *interval training*!

In 2008, English researchers published a study on the effects of intense sprint training on an exercise bike and its relationship to GH levels (137). The study revealed that a single 30-second, all-out sprint resulted in enormous surges in GH levels. However, with each additional sprint, the response became more blunted due to a negative feedback loop, possibly involving elevated fats in the bloodstream. Several important conclusions can be drawn from this study:

1. When doing interval training, fewer intervals may provide the same results as higher volumes.
2. The consumption of fat and/or carbohydrates prior to exercise may blunt the GH response, however refined the training protocol is.

Sprint interval training, whether on a bike, a treadmill or in a pool, is becoming increasingly popular for a number of reasons. When studies have compared sprint training with regular, continuous training, there have been similar improvements in cardiovascular fitness, as well as other biological functions. This may not seem significant, but when you factor in training time, it is nothing short of incredible. A commonly studied sprint interval training model consists of four to six 30-second, all-out sprint efforts, interspersed with four minutes of recovery in a single session. This means that with an extended warm-up and cool-down, the total training duration is in the region of 20 to 30 minutes per session.

In the last few years, there have been several studies proposing that even shorter sessions (≤10 min) are equally effective. For example, a Canadian research team recently published a peer-reviewed research article on three minutes of all-out sprint training per week (138). The six-week protocol involved only three 20-second, all-out sprints during a 10-minute training session, including warm-up and cool-down. Incredibly, the programme improved cardiorespiratory fitness by an average of 12%, lowered average blood pressure, and reduced 24-hour average blood glucose concentrations.

In 2016, a research article compared the effects of continuous, moderate-intensity aerobic training to high-intensity interval training. The study (139) divided 27 men into three groups: a control group, a continuous aerobic exercise group, and a high-intensity interval training group.

The interval protocol consisted of three 20-second, all-out cycling efforts (~500W), separated by 2 minutes of low-intensity cycling (only 50W). The continuous aerobic training protocol consisted of 45 minutes of cycling at ~70% of maximum heart rate. A 2-minute warm-up and 3-minute cool-down at 50W were included for both groups, resulting in 10- and 50-minute sessions for interval training and continuous training, respectively.

The 12-week protocol monitored weight, body fat percentage, body mass index, insulin, glucose, and other important health indicators. The findings showed that a total of 30 minutes per week of interval training is as effective as 150 minutes per week of continuous moderate-intensity training in increasing insulin sensitivity, cardiorespiratory fitness, and other important physical performance aspects, such as skeletal muscle mitochondrial[5] content.

However, the surprising finding was that interval training is more effective in reducing body weight and body fat percentage, despite the fact that training time was a fraction of that of the continuous training. The proposed mechanism is the dramatic increase in GH output that occurs in response to high-intensity exercise.

In summary, stress hormones are associated with a decline in GH levels, thereby impacting almost every facet of our physical integrity, functionality and health. Fortunately, there are many modalities we can incorporate into our daily lives to restore, and even increase natural GH levels. Exercise is a particularly potent stimulus, but needs to be highly specific.

The following protocols may be an effective tool in elevating GH levels.

Aerobic exercise

- Maximal effort (85–100%) sprint training for 20 to 30 seconds followed by 1 to 2 minutes of recovery, repeated 3 to 10 times[6]
- High-effort (±75% maximum heart rate) aerobic exercise for 10 minutes or longer
- Moderate intensity aerobic exercise (50–70% maximum heart rate) for periods exceeding two hours

Resistance training exercise

- Do exercises that target large muscle groups or have combined movements, such as squat and press, or step-up and curls
- Ensure moderate loads with a maximum of 10 repetitions
- Use a mini-circuit format
- Maintain short rest periods (less than a minute) between exercises or circuits
- A high amount of work must be performed in a short period of time

Go outdoors

The winter months are typically associated with reduced productivity and mental acuity, low motivation and, in some, a depressed state of mind. Frequently the antidote – a few days in a warm, sunny environment – is able to transform us back into the best version of ourselves. Remarkably, this enhanced state of cognitive and emotional well-being remains for weeks following our return home. Although this may appear isolated and nothing more than a personal experience, numerous studies reliably show seasonality in brain functionality and integrity. The reason for this has to do with a reduction in serotonin and BDNF levels that typically accompanies the winter months.

By virtue of the relationship between serotonin, BDNF and cognitive and emotional integrity, chronic stress can be compared to a protracted winter, limiting our potential in many areas of life.

Moderate sunlight exposure can effectively restore biological balance, both physically and cognitively during and after periods of chronic stress. The reason is multifactorial and involves several complex processes which, according to Harvard researchers (140), include elevations in beta-endorphins. Beta-endorphins are neurochemicals that promote a feeling of well-being, super-charge the immune system, relieve pain, promote relaxation, and even facilitate the specialisation of cells.

Additionally, sunlight exposure enhances the functionality of our DNA. In a 2015 study (141), researchers led by John Todd at Cambridge University evaluated blood and tissue samples from 16 000 people living in various regions of the world. The study aimed to identify the seasonal differences[7] in human health profiles. The researchers discovered that sunlight exposure influences the behaviour of over 5 136 genes (~23% of our gene pool), many of which have been shown to have a major influence on our health, specifically pertaining to inflammatory regulation. Considering that stress is associated with dysregulation of immune behaviours, these insights could prove immeasurably valuable in terms of restoring health during and after periods of chronic stress.

Moreover, sunlight has the potential to significantly lower the risk of developing cardiovascular issues, including heart attack and stroke, which are typically associated with chronic stress. In a recent study (142), a team of researchers from Edinburgh and Southampton universities showed that when the skin is exposed to ultraviolet (UV) radiation from the sun, nitrite and nitrate reserves found in the upper epidermis[8] are converted into nitric oxide gas. This gas then enters into the circulatory system, where it promotes dilation of our blood vessels, lowering blood pressure and enhancing functionality of the cardiovascular system.

The cardiovascular system is not the only system to benefit from the infusion of nitric oxide gas into the bloodstream. According to a 2016 review article by Dutch researchers (143), nitric oxide mobilisation through UV exposure is also associated with better weight control, improved glucose tolerance and lowered insulin resistance – all key factors influenced by chronic stress.

This may explain why Dr Pelle Lindqvist and other researchers at the Karolinska Institute have, perhaps controversially, warned against complete sun avoidance, comparing it with the dangers of smoking (144). This statement comes off the back of a 20-year study following the sunbathing habits of nearly 30 000 Swedish women. The study, published in the *Journal of Internal Medicine,* showed that avid sunbathers had a significantly lower risk of death from cardiovascular disease and other conditions that were not related to cancer. The study also showed that those who experienced modest sun exposure had a 40% lower risk of all-cause mortality than those who avoided the sun completely.

The evidence clearly shows that chronic stress is associated with a dysregulation of immune behaviours, manifesting in either immuno-suppression or, conversely, hyperactivity and autoimmune-related health disorders. Sunlight exposure can be extremely helpful in this regard.

According to Professor Gerald Ahern of the Department of Pharmacology and Physiology at Georgetown University, modest sunlight exposure lowers susceptibility to many illnesses. There are numerous mechanisms that drive this enhanced level of functionality. For example, Dr Ahern and his team found that low levels of blue light[9] energise specialised immune cells (T-cells) on the surface of the body, creating robust movement and enhanced activity, thereby offering improved protection from airborne viruses and pathogens (145). This action can be highly advantageous in stress-induced immune compromise.

Incredibly, while immune activity increases on the surface of the body, the inverse pattern occurs inside the body. A 2015 study (146) published in the journal *Archives of Biochemistry and Biophysics* showed that UV radiation was able to control various immune and inflammatory processes in the body, offering considerable protection from various autoimmune conditions.

Although sunlight positively influences the cardiovascular and immune systems, and positively enhances many metabolic processes, in the context of chronic stress, the greatest benefit derived from modest sunlight exposure is unquestionably in the realm of emotional and cognitive integrity. The reason lies in sunlight's direct effect on BDNF and serotonin.

A 2012 research article (147) published in the *Public Library of Science* showed a pronounced seasonal variation in serum (blood) BDNF concentrations with increasing levels in the spring-summer period, and decreasing concentrations in the autumn-winter period. This peer-reviewed Dutch study of 2 851 people found that the principal trigger in the rise in BDNF secretion rates is related to the number of sunlight hours in a day. Results of the study show that there is a significant difference between BDNF levels at the end of winter compared with the end of summer.

Not only does sunlight exposure influence BDNF levels, it also has a profound effect on serotonin[10] production. This is extremely advantageous because serotonin levels are compromised by the elevated cortisol levels that result from chronic stress.

The mechanism by which serotonin production is elevated by sunlight appears to be through an increase in the body's vitamin D[11] status. Vitamin D can be derived from a variety of sources; however sunlight exposure, in particular the UVB portion of sunlight, is the most effective means of increasing biological levels.

According to Dr Michael Horlick, an endocrinologist who has authored over 400 publications on vitamin D, this vitamin influences more than 80 metabolic processes. Additionally, Horlick attributes vitamin D to the control of almost 2 000 genes, many of which control cell growth, immune function, blood sugar stabilisation, and proper brain, heart and muscle function.

One of the most profound studies (148) on serotonin and its relationship to vitamin D status was published in 2014 in the *Journal of the Federation of American Societies for Experimental Biology*. The researchers from the Nutrition and Metabolism Center at the Children's Hospital Oakland Research Institute presented evidence showing that vitamin D activates the primary gene (TPH2) that is responsible for the production of serotonin, thereby affecting concentrations in the brain and body.[12]

Proceed with caution!

To optimise your levels of vitamin D through sunlight exposure, you need to consider:

- time of day
- length of time in the sun
- sunscreen
- skin type
- altitude
- latitude, and
- time of year.

Although modest sunlight exposure may offer significant health protection during periods of chronic stress, and several world-renowned researchers are calling insufficient sun exposure an emerging health problem (149), it is important to be mindful that sun exposure can be dangerous, especially in excess.

Most of the scientific literature still leans towards the risks, so warnings on the dangers of sun exposure should be heeded.

For a balanced perspective, speak to your dermatologist or doctor, as sun exposure guidance should be tailored to the individual. Factors such as age, skin type, history of skin and other cancers, current medical conditions and medications should always influence health practices.

Intermittent fasting and caloric restriction for a stronger body and mind

Intermittent fasting

Intermittent fasting is a method of caloric restriction where meal frequency is reduced to allow a 16- to 24-hour period when little or no food is consumed. This state produces numerous positive biological and metabolic shifts, which include decreased triglycerides (fats), lowered blood pressure, reduced insulin and greater insulin sensitivity. Additionally, intermittent fasting promotes genetic up-regulation[13] of certain genes, which promotes DNA repair and antioxidant activity, reduces inflammation, fights cancer cells and protects the body from stress. Intermittent fasting also elevates BDNF and GH.

Numerous studies have reliably shown considerable elevations in BDNF concentrations after periods of intermittent fasting or caloric restriction. A study by Japanese researchers (150) showed that alternate-day intermittent fasting increased BDNF levels by over 500% within a six-week period. The aim of the study was to assess the mechanism underlying the association between intermittent fasting and improved recovery odds in those who had suffered heart failure. While numerous contributing factors were identified, the researchers believe that the dramatic rise in BDNF was largely responsible for the improved health outcomes.

The question is, what does the heart have to do with the brain? The answer is, *everything*! As you know from the discussion on controlled breathing, the heart is actually a mini-brain containing one of the highest concentrations of neurons outside the executive brain (>40 000). This means that the regenerative processes of the heart depend on many of the same signalling proteins that are required in the promotion of brain integrity and development.

The study also shows that BDNF can offer tremendous cardiovascular protection. Since both the cardiovascular and nervous systems are severely compromised in response to chronic stress, intermittent fasting can be highly advantageous in the promotion of overall stress resilience, and the restoration of health after periods of chronic stress.

Not only does regular intermittent fasting raise BDNF levels, a single fast can have the same effect. A team of Canadian researchers (151) found that a single 48-hour fast elevated BDNF levels by a factor of 3.5!

Another study, published in the *Journal of Clinical Endocrinology & Metabolism* (152), found that two days of fasting increased the 24-hour production rate of growth hormone by 500%. For many, the mere thought of two days of food deprivation is in itself stress provoking. Fortunately, a fast of this duration is not necessary to elevate growth hormone secretion. GH levels are also positively influenced by shorter fasts. Several recent studies by Dr Benjamin Horne, Director of Cardiovascular and Genetic Epidemiology at the Intermountain Medical Center Heart Institute have shown that during 24-hour fasting periods, GH levels can increase by 1 300% in women and by 2 000% in men (153).

Several other markers of metabolic, cardiovascular and general health are also up-regulated in response to a 24-hour period of food abstinence. In a 2013 randomised crossover trial, 30 participants were assigned to a fasting group (water only) or a normal eating group for a period of 24 hours (154). Several health biomarkers were measured and evaluated. The data showed that the one-day fasting intervention acutely increased GH, haemoglobin, red blood cell count and HDLC,[14] while at the same time decreasing triglycerides and weight when compared with a day of usual eating.

With the plethora of health benefits associated with short fasts (16 to 24 hours) you might be motivated to do longer or even more frequent fasts with the intention of achieving greater results. Interestingly, longer fasts or increased frequency may not offer the same health returns in terms of cognitive and physical augmentation. According to a review by researchers from the Johns Hopkins University School of Medicine and the University of Southern California (155), three to five days of fasting results in a decline in several biological systems[15] as the body begins to preserve its precious resources. Although certain health conditions and diseases, such as cancer, may be effectively managed and even prevented by this slow-down, it is unlikely to be of value for those experiencing chronic stress. As in many health choices, there is a fine balance between dose and effect. Within this space, *moderation* offers the greatest returns.

Intermittent fasting (16/8 method)

Warning: This method should not be adopted by anyone who is pregnant or breastfeeding, hypoglycaemic, diabetic, has a history of eating disorders, suffers from adrenal fatigue, has low blood pressure or who suffers from any medical condition for which irregular meals are contra-indicated.

The core concept in intermittent fasting is to limit food consumption to a 6- to 8-hour window during the day. This can easily be achieved by skipping dinner or breakfast. For example, have dinner at 8 pm, then eat lunch the next day at 12 pm or 1 pm. Alternatively, the last meal of the day can be lunch at 1 pm or 2 pm followed by breakfast the next morning at 6 am or 7 am. It is suggested that women perform slightly shorter fasts, limiting food consumption to a 9- to 10-hour window – in other words, a 14- to 15-hour fast.

Water, herbal teas and even coffee in moderation are permitted during the fasts provided they are not caloric.[16]

Perform this intermittent fasting one to three days per week.

Warning: Other fasting protocols that are more extreme, for example fasts for longer than 36 hours or consuming less than 600 calories per day several days in a row are not recommended. These protocols place undue strain on the body and can affect your appetite centres, which can lead to binging and cravings for caloric foods.

Caloric restriction

For those who are unable[17] or unwilling to introduce intermittent fasting into their weekly or monthly routines, caloric restriction can offer similar benefits and is considerably easier to incorporate. Caloric restriction requires that you reduce your intake of food by a certain percentage (8–40%) over an extended period of time.

Researchers at Princeton and Johns Hopkins Universities (156) investigated the effects of extended caloric restriction on BDNF levels in mice. They found that by restricting food intake by 40% for almost twelve weeks, the expression of BDNF in key regions of the brain that control memory and learning had increased, as had the overall volume of brain tissue.

Other studies suggest that even smaller long-term adjustments to food intake can increase BDNF expression. A 2015 study published in the *International Heart Journal* (157) found that a 30% caloric restriction over a 28-day period increased BDNF, decreased oxidative stress, and improved memory and learning performance in rats with metabolic syndrome.

Although many of the studies on intermittent fasting and caloric restriction have been performed on animals, it is widely believed that they have very similar effects on humans.

Despite the numerous positive shifts in biological behaviour that support stress resilience, long periods of severe caloric restriction are neither practical nor recommended. The reason is that caloric restrictions of 30 to 60% over protracted periods can create significant nutrient deficiencies and ultimately lead to a decline in overall health, especially in older populations.

Fortunately, the research does suggest a middle ground, where caloric restrictions can be implemented for long periods of time without strain or ill effects. A study published in the *Journal of Applied Physiology* (158) showed that an 8% reduction in caloric intake is able to provide enormous life extension and health benefits, with little or no risk of nutrient deficiencies.

Other long-term data shows that an 11% caloric restriction can have extremely positive effects on disease profiles, lifespan and functionality. A recent study published in *Current Opinion in Clinical Nutrition and Metabolic Care* (159) investigated the health profiles of Japanese nationals living on Okinawa Island. This remarkable population has among the highest longevity in the world – five times as many centenarians than other industrialised countries – and has some of the lowest rates of cancer, heart disease and disability. In fact, Okinawans have almost a decade of additional disability-free life expectancy when compared with Americans and other industrialised nations.

Researchers believe that caloric restriction to the extent of 11% and selective food choices are largely responsible for this phenomenon, rather than genetics.

There are various protocols that can promote elevated BDNF and other biologically protective responses; however when under chronic stress and in a state of elevated cortisol, caloric restriction rather than intermittent fasting may be less demanding, both psychologically and physically.

In recent years, concerns have been raised about the long-term impact of intermittent fasting and caloric restriction on the hormonal system, cortisol levels and inflammatory markers.

Whereas several older animal studies have shown that protracted caloric restriction decreases GH and increases corticosterone[18] levels by 30 to 50% (160, 161), more recent research, including randomised clinical trials and cross-sectional observational studies, indicates that caloric restriction for periods of 6 to 12 months does not result in elevations of cortisol, nor does it alter GH profiles, provided that protein intakes are maintained throughout the dietary intervention (162, 163, 164).

Athletes are a unique group for whom caloric restriction or intermittent fasting may *not* be advantageous during periods of chronic stress due to their rigorous physical demands. New research has shown that the combined effect of high-intensity training or intense competition with periods of significant caloric restriction can trigger the stress axis, resulting in increased inflammation, elevated cortisol and reduced hormonal integrity.

For example, a 2015 study on combative[19] athletes published in *Oxidative*

Medicine and Cellular Longevity found that while GH levels were raised in response to the combination of caloric restriction and intense sports training, so too were inflammatory markers (IL-6, TNF-α) and cortisol (165). The study also revealed a marked decline in performance, weight and testosterone levels.

Both intermittent fasting and moderate caloric restriction can be beneficial in promoting stress resilience and health across multiple domains. If you suffer from certain medical conditions, such as adrenal fatigue, kidney dysfunction or diabetes; have a history of eating disorders or train exceptionally hard on a regular basis, this is **not** suited to you! It is still strongly advised that you consult with your doctor prior to implementing dietary changes, especially if you have an underlying medical condition or pre-existing health issues.

I have provided several examples of popular and commonly prescribed protocols. Try to select one that best suits your lifestyle and preferences.

Caloric restriction protocols

Large restriction
- Restrict calorie intake by 60% while maintaining high nutrient intake – vitamins, minerals, antioxidants, and so on.
- Perform only one to two days per week.

Medium restriction
- Restrict calorie intake by 30 to 40% while maintaining high nutrient intake – vitamins, minerals, antioxidants, and so on.
- Perform a maximum of two to four days per week.

Moderate restriction
- Restrict calorie intake by 15% while maintaining high nutrient intake – vitamins, minerals, antioxidants, and so on.
- Perform five to six days per week.

Caloric deficit protocol

The 25% reduction

This is typically a six-month protocol involving a 25% reduction in overall energy balance. The adjustment is created by a 12.5% increase in energy expenditure through daily exercise, combined with a 12.5% reduction in calorie intake.

FOOD AND SUPPLEMENTS IN THE FIGHT AGAINST CHRONIC STRESS

Of particular interest in the pharmaceutical and nutraceutical sectors are caloric restriction mimetics.[20] These compounds provide the physiological benefit of caloric restriction without actually restricting calories. Many of these nutrients or foods have been shown to trigger significant elevations in BDNF and serotonin, as well as cause substantial reductions in stress hormones. Additionally, research shows that they enable important genes[21] and biological processes (autophagy[22]) that lengthen health span[23] and facilitate maximum functionality. Some of these foods and nutrients include resveratrol, sweet potato-based compounds, marine-based oils, carotenoid-rich foods, curcumin (found in turmeric) and various flavonoids[24] (especially from soy foods).

Curcumin

Curcumin is a potent caloric restriction mimetic that has been used in India and China to manage stress, anxiety and depression for more than 2 000 years. It is the active ingredient in the spice we know as turmeric.[25]

The use of curcumin as a health-promoting supplement has exploded in recent years.

General health benefits

Not only does curcumin offer a strong direct and indirect defence against chronic stress, it also offers protection from several of the more common health ailments that are becoming more prevalent in industrialised nations. According to an article published in the *Indian Journal of Pharmaceutical Sciences* (166), curcumin may provide protection against many cancers, as well as autoimmune, cardiovascular and neurological diseases, in addition to protecting key organ systems from toxicity.

Curcumin protects against stress-induced depression and declines in BDNF

Curcumin has the ability to negate many of the negative effects of chronic stress, particularly stabilising BDNF levels in the brain. In 2014, researchers at the Shandong University School of Medicine in China published one of the first *in vivo*[26] studies (167) on the effects of curcumin on stress, altered behaviour and the structural integrity of the brain.

The six-week animal study showed that in a simulated stress model, BDNF levels declined by more than 40%. The decline in BDNF was particularly apparent in the brain's fear modulator, the amygdala.[27] As mentioned previously, the long-term impact of lowered BDNF would certainly predispose the brain to a significant decline in structural integrity and functional capabilities. Remarkably, the study showed that the group given curcumin prior to and during the stress simulations had almost no decline in circulating BDNF. According to the authors, the results suggest that long-term administration of curcumin may offer the brain complete protection from the adverse effects of chronic stress. Additionally, curcumin administration negated stress-induced depressive-like behaviour to such an extent that it paralleled common antidepressant medications, without the side effects or danger of dependency. According to the researchers:

Given these results, pre-treatment with curcumin has a potential function as a novel antidepressant agent for the amelioration of depression.

Not only may curcumin provide protection for the brain during periods of chronic stress, it has also been shown to neutralise some of the adverse effects of the stress hormones themselves. In 2011, the journal *Neuroscience Letters* published a study (168) showing that administration of synthetic stress hormones (corticosteroids) for a period of three weeks resulted in depression and lowered BDNF levels in the hippocampus and frontal cortex.[28] Yet again, when curcumin was administered under these biologically hostile conditions (copious amounts of cortisone), BDNF levels were stabilised and depression was averted, despite ongoing exposure.

Supporting these studies, recent evidence suggests that curcumin may even modulate the entire stress response. The evidence for this comes from a Chinese study (169) on rats that were continuously exposed to stress simulations for four weeks. The researchers found that by administering curcumin during the stressful period, the rats were able to moderate their stress responses to the same extent that the antidepressant Prozac would, reducing the incidence of hyper-emotional states and irrationality without any of the potential side effects.

Curcumin optimises neurochemical balance

Not only does chronic stress negatively affect the structural integrity of the brain, it also affects its performance. This is especially true in terms of memory, cognition, attention, focus, learning, problem-solving, sleep and behaviour. Many of these cognitive attributes, which are critical to success in life, are driven by the neurotransmitters serotonin, dopamine, gluta-mate[29] and norepinephrine. Chronic stress is known to cause significant alterations in the balance of these neurotransmitters leading to a variety of emotional and cognitive disorders. Remarkably, according to an Australian review of the literature in 2012 (170), curcumin has been shown to pro-mote optimal neurochemical integrity and balance in a variety of research settings.

Challenges with supplementation

One of the principal issues with curcumin supplementation is that it is poorly absorbed on its own. According to *BMC Complementary and Alternative Medicine*, extreme doses of up to 8 000 mg of curcumin can sometimes fail to significantly increase blood levels (171).

The key is to combine curcumin with compounds that enhance its bioavailability and absorption. Japanese researchers found that combining curcumin with piperidine, which is found in black pepper, increases bio-availability more than 20-fold (172).

Also, curcumin combined with phospholipids found in foods such as eggs, soy, peanuts, dairy products, organ meats and some seeds, amplifies the bioavailability. A randomised, double-blind, crossover human study published in the *Journal of Natural Products* (173) found that by combining curcumin with a phospholipid formulation known as Meriva, curcumin bioavailability increased 29-fold!

One of the most exciting developments is the entry of theracurmin into the marketplace. Theracurmin is a modified version of curcumin that has a smaller particle size and is more soluble. Japanese researchers found that the bioavailability of curcumin in the theracurmin preparation increased 27-fold in humans (172). All indications are that a newer generation of the product is making its debut in 2018, which is believed to have even greater bioavailability.

Choosing a product

Throughout the world, nutraceuticals are big business! Despite this, the supplement industry appears to be poorly regulated, making it a challenge to choose a safe and effective product. Always opt for long-standing, reputable companies that advertise stringent regulatory standards and quality assurance.

Food sources

Turmeric is the principal food source containing curcumin. It is a yellow spice typically used in Indian, Southeast Asian and Middle Eastern cuisine. According to *Phytochemical Analysis: PCA* (174), curcuminoids[30] make up about 2 to 9% of turmeric. Curcumin happens to be the most abundant curcuminoid in turmeric (75%). Turmeric also contains important minerals, such as manganese, potassium, magnesium and iron, as well as fibre, vitamin B6 and vitamin C. Turmeric is widely regarded as perfectly safe, even in high doses.

Pregnancy and lactation

Because the safety of curcumin during pregnancy and lactation has not been established, supplements (not foods) containing curcumin should be avoided, to be on the safe side.

Toxicity and side effects

To date, there are a limited number of human trials investigating curcumin toxicity, but two human studies (175, 176) have found that even huge doses of up to 12 g appear safe and well tolerated. This said, I would always stick to lower dosages because, as a recent Chinese study (177) showed, overdosing animals for extended periods of time resulted in liver damage, as would overdosing on any supplement.

Some minor side effects can arise from higher doses (4–12 g per day), which may include nausea, headache, reflux, bloating, and even a minor rash.

Medication interactions

Not to be taken with anti-platelet or anticoagulant medications
A Danish study (176) found that curcumin could inhibit platelet aggregation,[31] suggesting that supplementation would increase the risk of bleeding or bruising in people taking anticoagulant or anti-platelet medications.

Many chronic medications may be compromised by curcumin supplementation
There is also research indicating that curcumin may interfere with the bioavailability of many medications by speeding up their metabolism through the activation of certain liver enzymes.

Resveratrol

Resveratrol is a plant compound that acts much like an antioxidant. There are over 70 known natural food sources of resveratrol, some of which include red wine, grapes, blueberries, blackberries, pistachios and peanuts.

Resveratrol is a phytoalexin. These chemicals are characterised by their ability to inhibit the progress of certain infections in plants. They do this by accumulating in the plant in response to adverse conditions, such as parasites, fungal infection, UV radiation, chemical exposure, and other such demanding factors.

Resveratrol's health-promoting properties
Like curcumin, resveratrol is a caloric restriction mimetic that has been used in Eastern medicine for over 2 000 years. Because it is able to interact with a large array of biomolecules, resveratrol has many health-promoting properties.

According to researchers at the University of Valencia (178), resveratrol has anti-carcinogenic properties, can inhibit blood clotting, is a powerful antioxidant, and has anti-ageing, anti-frailty, anti-inflammatory and anti-allergenic properties. These beneficial biological effects have been extensively studied in both humans and animals.

Considering that chronic stress is associated with increased free radical formation, inflammation and accelerated ageing, resveratrol could be a very beneficial compound within the broader resilience model.

Resveratrol increases BDNF and lowers risk of stress-related psychological issues

Resveratrol has been found to positively alter both psychological and physiological responses to stress. A 2016 study by Chinese researchers (179) confirmed that five weeks of progressive stress caused a significant rise in stress hormones, lowered BDNF and induced depressive-like behaviour. However, the researchers also discovered that resveratrol negated all the negative responses attributed to stress, including the depressive state. Simply put, resveratrol offers broad-spectrum protection. According to the researchers:

> All of these effects of resveratrol were essentially identical to those observed with the established antidepressant, desipramine.

This was by no means an isolated study. In 2016, a team from Shandong University School of Medicine in China published a research report (179) that supported the 2016 study's findings, only this time the antidepressant comparison was with the famous fluoxetine (Prozac). The results showed that resveratrol administration for only three weeks, in contrast to five in the 2016 study, significantly reversed the stress-induced behavioural abnormalities (anxiety and depression) largely by up-regulating BDNF, as well as by promoting several positive cellular changes in the brain.

A study (180) published in *Behavioural Brain Research* investigated the effects of seven days of intravenous administration of resveratrol in rats, specifically looking at whether resveratrol administration may be associated with an increase in brain concentrations of BDNF. The researchers found that high doses of resveratrol caused the levels of BDNF in the hippocampus[32] to spike by 24% within a period of only a week.

Resveratrol lowers stress hormone responses

In 2013, another team of Chinese researchers (181) suggested that the underlying mechanism behind many of the positive effects of resveratrol in the context of chronic stress was actually stabilisation of the entire stress axis.

Chronic stress is typically associated with overreactivity of the stress axis resulting in a release of stress hormones that is often disproportionate to life's challenges. This study showed that resveratrol administration was able to normalise peripheral stress responses – that is, the stress hormone levels in the body – without influencing the hormonal state in the brain itself.

Resveratrol provides neurological protection

Resveratrol has come to the attention of neuroscientists in recent years because of its powerful neuroprotective actions and ability to activate the Sirtuins (SIRT) family member, SIRT1.[33]

The effects are so powerful that this plant compound is now considered an effective means of managing several complex brain disorders. According to a review article (182) entitled "Neuroprotective properties of resveratrol in different neurodegenerative disorders", resveratrol has been effective in managing Alzheimer's disease, ischaemic stroke, Parkinson's disease, Huntington's disease and epilepsy.

If resveratrol can be successful in the treatment of these ailments, you can only imagine the benefits that it could have for a chronically stressed brain. Moreover, not only does resveratrol benefit the brain by enhancing the expression of the SIRT1 family of proteins, it also positively influences two neurochemicals that are negatively impacted by chronic stress – serotonin and norepinephrine. Collectively, these neurochemicals influence sleep, mood, behaviour, anxiety, depression, cognition, and several other key neurological processes.

In 2010, *European Neuropsychopharmacology* published a study (183) showing that, in animals, resveratrol produced a significant increase in serotonin and noradrenalin as measured by both behavioural models and neurochemical assessments.

Side effects and precautions

Resveratrol has a similar structure to oestrogen. Although not as similar as many other bioflavonoids,[34] it is similar enough to potentially interfere with normal oestrogen metabolism. While researchers have concerns about certain forms of cancer, menstrual irregularities and other oestrogen-related biological functions, not much evidence of this has surfaced yet. Although it is certainly worth being cautious, the current body of evidence is in favour of resveratrol's anti-carcinogenic effects. It is best to speak to your doctor to assess whether this supplement is right for you.

Toxicity

Resveratrol is not known to be toxic or to cause significant adverse effects in humans, but there haven't been many controlled clinical trials to date.

According to researchers from the Department of Cancer Studies and Molecular Medicine at the University of Leicester (184), large doses of up to 5 g have been taken with no side effects, apart from some intestinal upset and occasional nausea. However, extended periods of doses exceeding 1 g per day might result in nausea, abdominal pain, flatulence and diarrhoea.

Pregnancy and lactation

The safety of resveratrol during pregnancy and lactation has not been established, so to be on the safe side, avoid supplements (not foods) containing resveratrol.

Medication interactions

Because resveratrol strongly affects numerous biological systems, it may have interactions with common medications.

Avoid if you are taking anti-coagulant, anti-platelet and anti-inflammatory medications

High doses of supplemented resveratrol could increase the risk of bruising and bleeding when taken with anti-coagulant and anti-platelet drugs, as well as non-steroidal anti-inflammatories.

Avoid if you are on chronic medications

Resveratrol could reduce the metabolic clearance of certain medications, increasing the risk of their toxicity. These medications include antihistamines, immunosuppressants, statins and calcium channel blockers.

Conversely, a study published in *Cancer Prevention Research* (185) investigating the effect of pharmacological doses of resveratrol on drug- and carcinogen-metabolising enzymes found that resveratrol induced the expression and activity of an enzyme called CYP1A2, which promotes the metabolism of several medications, including paracetamol and several antidepressants. This essentially means that these medications could be cleared out of the system too rapidly, possibly lowering their circulating concentrations to below therapeutic levels.

Despite the wealth of recent evidence, research in this area still has a long way to go, as there are a limited number of studies looking at the long-term effects of resveratrol supplementation on health outcomes in humans.

Resveratrol supplementation

One of the issues with resveratrol supplementation is that only a small percentage is able to enter the bloodstream when orally ingested. Because of this, *you need to time your intake perfectly*. Remarkably, there is a circadian rhythm[35] to resveratrol absorption. Portuguese researchers (186) found that the concentration of resveratrol in the blood is more dose-efficient (more bioavailable) in the morning, when compared to the evening. This shows a potential relationship to cortisol.

Another challenge with resveratrol supplementation is the fact that there also appears to be variation between individuals within the context of bioavailability, because some people absorb it better than others. However, this is more magnified with higher doses. This makes it challenging to prescribe the optimal dosage.

Taken on an empty stomach or with meals?

Research shows that concurrent food intake has little or no impact on bioavailability, although the point at which resveratrol levels peak in the bloodstream may be a little delayed (187), especially with fatty meals (>45 g fat).

Choosing a product and dosage

Only choose resveratrol products from long-standing, reputable companies that advertise stringent regulatory standards and quality assurance.

Ideally, purchase micro-ionised resveratrol as it has 3.6 times the bioavailability of other forms. The recommended dose is 100–500 mg per day. However, doses up to 1 500 mg have been used safely and effectively. Just remember, when it comes to most supplements, less is always more!

Foods containing resveratrol

Even though natural foods contain significantly lower amounts of resveratrol, in many respects they are preferable to nutraceuticals because they contain a spectrum of compounds that work synergistically[36] to dramatically increase bioavailability. Of course, organic sources are best as they are free of pesticides and contain a more enriched nutrient profile.

The best natural food sources of resveratrol include red grapes; grape juice; peanuts; pistachios; cocoa; berries of the *Vaccinium* species, including blueberries, bilberries and cranberries; and most notably, red wine.

What makes red wine a particularly good source of resveratrol is the fact that the alcohol produced in the fermentation process facilitates resveratrol's solubility, and thus its extraction. The only drawback is that you have to consume a fair amount to get sufficient amounts of resveratrol.

And as you will read later, alcohol and stress are not the best combination!

Omega-3 fatty acids

Marine-derived omega-3 fatty acids are believed to be the single most important nutrient complex in the human diet, contributing to numerous essential biological functions. Obtaining adequate amounts of omega-3 fatty acids is becoming increasingly more difficult in light of the current trend in modern dietary habits. There are two reasons for this:

- the best sources are not modern-day food preferences (mackerel, herring, sardines, grass-fed meat, walnuts), and
- the levels of omega-3 fatty acids in our food are steadily declining.

According to an article published in *Experimental Biology and Medicine* (188), the ratio between marine-based omega-3 (marine-based oils) and omega-6 (plant-based oils) in our ancestral diet was in the region of 1:1. This historic ratio established our genetic patterns and promoted optimal functioning of our nervous, cardiovascular and immune systems. Today, this ratio has been drastically distorted in that the standard American diet tends to have a ratio highly favouring omega-6 fatty acids, in the region of 1:20! The modern European diet, specifically in the UK, is not significantly better. According to researchers at the Food and Health Research Centre at King's College in London (189), the dietary ratio of omega-3 to omega-6 fatty acids in many parts of Europe is around 1:15. Research has reliably shown that these abnormal proportions promote the development of many diseases, including cardiovascular disease, cancer, and inflammatory and autoimmune diseases.

The best evidence for the positive effects of marine-derived omega-3 fatty acids on human health is seen in certain sectors of the Japanese population. It is well established that Japan has the greatest overall longevity in the world, together with some of the lowest rates of cardiovascular disease and cancers. According to a study published in *The American Journal of Clinical Nutrition* (190), the ratio of omega-3 to omega-6 fatty acids in Japan is 1:4. It is not surprising that other regions of the world, such as the Mediterranean and Scandinavia have exceptional longevity and low rates of chronic diseases, since they share the same trend with the Japanese – higher omega-3 to omega-6 ratios.

An extensive Harvard study (191) investigating the modifiable factors[37] responsible for premature or preventable deaths in the US found that omega-3 fatty acid deficiencies account for over 100 000 deaths each year.

Although plant-derived omega-3 fatty acids offer good health benefits, the composition is somewhat different from marine sources, and requires an extensive conversion through enzymatic channels. Linseed or flax seed, pumpkin seed, walnuts, chia seeds, soya and green leafy vegetables are high in omega-3 and alpha-linoleic acid (ALA).

Most of the biological benefits are derived from eicosapentaenoic acid (EPA) and docosahexaenoic acid (DHA) omega-3 fatty acids, which are found exclusively in cold water fish. Interestingly, EPA and DHA are derived indirectly from marine algae and their availability is *increased* as they pass up the food chain, becoming highly concentrated in the flesh of marine fish, which include mackerel, salmon, tuna, sardines and herring.

If you are vegetarian or vegan or don't want to consume fish, you can purchase **marine algae supplements** to derive equal, if not greater, benefits.

Omega-3 fatty acids stabilise stress hormone output
Omega-3 fatty acids have a remarkable ability to normalise biological processes in a wide variety of settings. This has stirred a lot of interest in supplementation in the context of chronic stress. In 2003, French and Swiss researchers published a study (192) showing how omega-3 fatty acid supplementation can lower stress hormone responses to a perceived challenge. The study involved a

small group of participants who were monitored during two distinct periods, before and after three weeks of supplementation with 7.2 g fish oil per day, which is a fairly high dose.

On each occasion, the concentrations of stress hormones in the blood, energy expenditure and blood fats were monitored in basal conditions, followed by a 30-minute mental stress simulation and a 30-minute recovery period.

As expected, under normal conditions mental stress significantly increased heart rate, mean blood pressure and overall energy expenditure. Stress also increased adrenalin levels by more than 50%, cortisol by more than 30%, and fat concentrations in the bloodstream by more than 30%.

Incredibly, when the participants were retested following three weeks on a diet supplemented with omega-3 fatty acids, adrenalin, cortisol, energy expenditure and fatty acid concentrations in the bloodstream were all significantly blunted.

The researchers believed that supplementation with omega-3 fatty acids inhibits and/or stabilises the adrenal activation triggered by mental stress through unexplained effects on the brain.

New evidence is emerging showing that omega-3 fatty acid supplementation, especially when in combination with phosphatidylserine, is particularly effective in promoting biological stability in those with higher levels of chronic stress, as well as those who have a disrupted and/or dysfunctional stress response.[38]

Omega-3 fatty acids protect the brain cells from the damaging effects of cortisol

One of the most significant influences of omega-3 fatty acid supplementation is in supporting the structure and function of the brain during periods of chronic stress. It does this through a variety of mechanisms, one of which is by negating the effects of stress hormones (specifically cortisol) on brain tissue. A 2016 study published in the *International Journal of Neuropsychopharmacology* (193) showed that when brain cells from the frontal cortex[39] are exposed to corticotrophins[40] they become structurally compromised and die.

The interesting thing about the study was that 24 hours of corticotrophin exposure had no effect on brain cells, regardless of the amount. However, after 48 hours of stress hormone exposure, brain cells became damaged and structurally compromised. Incredibly, when the same kind of cells were treated with a specific dose of omega-3 fatty acids,[41] the fatty acid was absorbed into the brain cells, and both their integrity and numbers remained intact. Not only does this study show the value of omega-3 fatty acid intake in supporting the brain during periods of chronic stress, it also illustrates how resilient our brains are in the face of short bursts of stress.

Long-term administration of omega-3 fatty acids increases BDNF as well as brain size

Another mechanism by which omega-3 fatty acids protect our brains during times of stress is through the up-regulation of BDNF. In 2014, a team of researchers at the University of Berlin's Department of Neurology published a double-blind, randomised, interventional study (194) showing that ongoing supplementation with omega-3 fatty acids results in significant cognitive improvements in human subjects, largely through elevations in BDNF. The study involved 65 healthy subjects who were given either 2.2 g of fish oil or a placebo for a period of 26 weeks. A large range of tests were performed before and after the intervention, including cognitive performance and neuro-imaging.

The findings showed that the subjects who took omega-3 fatty acids exhibited an increase in brain mass in numerous regions of the brain, including the frontal, temporal, parietal and limbic areas. Additionally, cognition was markedly higher.

It appears that dose is everything! A 2008 Dutch, double-blind interventional study (195) of healthy, older subjects could not detect specific effects on cognitive functions after 26 weeks of supplementation. The difference in the studies appears to be dose. The Dutch study involved either a 400 mg or 1 800 mg dose per day, which was significantly lower than the German study.

Omega-3 fatty acids control inflammation at the source

The first wave of stress is associated with considerable immune activation and increased inflammation. Because many diseases have their origins in chronic[42] inflammation, it is important to restore stability within the body as quickly as possible.

Over the last four decades, both human and animal studies have demonstrated that omega-3 fatty acids can suppress inflammation and play a beneficial role in a variety of stress-induced inflammatory diseases.[43]

Until recently, the mechanism by which omega-3 fatty acids lower inflammation in the body was not fully understood. A collaborative study by Chinese and Swiss researchers (196) showed that omega-3 fatty acids inhibit the main protein, NLRP3 inflammasome, which is responsible for turning on the inflammatory response. What is incredible about omega-3 fatty acids is that they not only manage the effects of the inflammatory process; more importantly, they control it at source. The health implications of this mechanism in terms of chronic stress are enormous.

Omega-3 fatty acids influence our neurochemistry

Another positive influence of omega-3 fatty acids on stress resilience is in the area of serotonin. Dr Rhonda Patrick and Dr Bruce Ames of the Nutrition and Metabolism Center at the Children's Hospital Oakland Research Institute published a study (197) outlining the value of omega-3 fatty acids in serotonin functionality. The study showed that the release and uptake of serotonin in the brain is directly related to the levels of marine-derived omega-3 fatty acids.

Dietary sources

The best dietary sources of omega-3 fatty acids include salmon, sardines, mackerel, tuna and anchovies. However, you must take into account that a certain degree of contamination may be present in some fish species, especially farmed fish and large bottom feeders. In terms of public health and safety, researchers and scientists are most concerned about four groups of toxins: methylmercury, polychlorinated bisphenols, dioxins and organochlorines.

Of these contaminants, methylmercury is of primary concern. Firstly, WHO (198) considers methylmercury to be one of the top ten dangers to public health. According to WHO, even small amounts of this form of mercury can damage the nervous, immune and digestive systems, as well as the lungs, kidneys and eyes. Developing foetuses are particularly vulnerable; expectant mothers need to be hyper-vigilant and limit their exposure by avoiding certain species of fish.

Secondly, the Environmental Protection Agency (EPA)(199) asserts that exposure to methylmercury may result in visual disturbances, muscle weakness, poor coordination, and significant cognitive impairment, including loss of memory, poor attention, and loss of executive functions.

Warning: Amongst other things, ingestion of methylmercury can:

- damage your brain and nerves, causing cognitive impairment such as loss of memory and executive functions
- compromise your body's ability to fight infections and repair itself
- cause muscle weakness, poor coordination, visual disturbance, and
- damage your lungs and kidneys.

According to an article published in *Circulation* (200), when epidemiological studies investigating the effects of marine-derived omega-3 fatty acids showed weak findings or poor outcomes, it corresponded to an elevated intake of methylmercury. The reason for this is that mercury and omega-3 fatty acids are diametrically opposed in their effects on the body, especially in the brain.

The issue with mercury contamination is that it cannot be minimised or reduced through trimming the fat and skin, or even by draining the fat during the cooking process. Methylmercury does not bind to fat like other contaminants. Rather, methylmercury is bound to the muscle tissue and the cooking process may even solidify the mercury content.

According to a 2003 research article in *Environmental Health Perspectives* (201), 95% of the mercury found in fish will be absorbed and taken up by body tissues within a 48-hour period. What's most concerning is that researchers from the Division of Environmental and Occupational Epidemiology at the Michigan Department of Community Health (202) found that mercury remains in the adult body for at least 70 to 90 days. On top of that, regular consumption of contaminated seafood may cause accumulation of mercury in the body, especially when the rate of consumption exceeds the rate at which the body can eliminate it.[44]

Guidelines to optimise omega-3 intake and minimise mercury exposure

1. Eat 220 to 350 g of a variety of fish every week. This equates to roughly two or three small servings.
2. Choose fish that is known to be lower in mercury. The Council for Scientific and Industrial Research (CSIR) has recently published data on the concentrations of mercury found in fish species that are readily available in South Africa (203). The research provides advice on how many servings the public can safely consume.

According to Dr Brent Newman at the CSIR, the guidelines are as follows:

1. *Safest* (13–36 portions per month): sardines, German sea bream, west-coast sole, mackerel and Cape knife jaw
2. *Consume moderately* (4–10 portions per month): yellowtail, hake (cod), shad, rock cod, stumpnose, kob, dorado, angelfish, red roman and steenbras
3. *Limited consumption* (2–3 portions per month): Cape salmon, tuna, kingklip, mussel cracker, garrick, farmed salmon and jacopever
4. *Avoid* (<1 portion a month): swordfish and bluefin tuna

For those living in the northern hemisphere, information on the safety and consumption guidelines for local and regional fish species are available on the Food and Drug Administration (FDA) website.

> Before eating fish that you or others have caught from streams, rivers and lakes, pay attention to any fish advisories that apply to that body of water.

Safety of omega-3 fatty acid supplements

Although there have been concerns about the potential for marine-derived omega-3 fatty acid supplements to contain methylmercury or other known contaminants, several independent laboratory analyses in the US and around the world have found commercially available omega-3 fatty acid supplements to be free of these harmful compounds, with very few exceptions.

The best omega-3 fatty acids are those that come from sardines, mackerel and anchovies, and have been purified. Antarctic krill can also be a good option, but it is important to ensure that it is 100% organic and naturally extracted.

Simply put, there is little to no contamination in high-quality fish oil supplements.

The principal issue with fish oil supplements is oxidation during manufacturing and storage. Oxidation can make the oil rancid, causing discoloration and a pungent smell. The more concerning issue is that the free radicals that are formed through exposure to oxygen render the oil completely unfit for human consumption and are likely to result in an antagonistic response, namely poor health outcomes.

Even though oils are more environmentally sensitive[45] than capsules, there is a higher degree of transparency pertaining to the integrity of the oil. Smell, taste and colour are three elements that can alert you to a rancid and potentially toxic product. Capsules may disguise this, which is why I prefer the oil option, if you can tolerate the taste.

The general consensus in the health sector is that the best fish oil supplements provide at least 1 000 mg of EPA and DHA per serving, are sustainably sourced, and are certified by third-party labs to ensure potency, purity and freshness.

Dosage

The US Institute of Medicine does not have guidelines for the intake of EPA and DHA at this time. However, the European Food Safety Authority (EFSA) has proposed adequate intakes for all forms of omega-3 fatty acids (plant- and marine-derived). The EFSA recommends an ALA intake[46] of 0.5% of total energy and 250 mg per day for marine-derived EPA plus DHA.

The World Health Organization recommends that daily omega-3 fatty acid intake constitutes 0.5 to 2% of total energy consumption from either marine or plant sources.

The International Society for the Study of Fatty Acids and Lipids (ISSFAL) recommends 0.7% of total caloric intake from plant sources, and a minimum of 500 mg per day of EPA plus DHA from marine sources for healthy adults.

Multivitamins

Dietary supplements have become increasingly popular. Manufacturers and suppliers promote nutraceuticals as the ultimate stress solution, as evidenced by the plethora of specialised formulations that have flooded the market in recent years. Products claiming to reduce stress-induced fatigue, anxiety, burnout, depression, adrenal fatigue and thyroid dysfunction are now commonplace in pharmacies and health stores throughout the developed world.

While nutrient deficiencies are certainly becoming more prevalent for many reasons,[47] the notion that the resolution of stress-induced health issues and enhancement of physical resilience can be achieved by super-dosing with a single nutrient or the consumption of a specialised dietary product is completely naive. Yet it does appeal to a broader cross-section of society – a 'quick fix' has great appeal nowadays.

Don't get me wrong, supplements play a very important role in stress management and resilience. However, we have to consider that dietary supplements, however beneficial, are merely tools that need to be incorporated into the larger whole that is personal health and resilience.

Multivitamins are commonly used to manage a variety of stress-related health issues such as general fatigue, burnout, and even general, stress-induced ill health. These micronutrient formulas are so in demand that, according to the *Nutrition Business Journal* (204), the annual revenue from multivitamin sales alone currently exceeds $5.8 billion. According to Grand View Research, by 2024 the global dietary supplement industry will be worth over $278 billion annually.

With such popularity, you would expect an abundance of research supporting multivitamin use in the context of stress management and resilience. Yet, despite their widespread demand and popularity, there are only a handful of high-quality, controlled trials that directly investigate the potential relationship between stress and multivitamin supplementation.

So what does the science say? Is this demand justified?

The answer is *yes*! The science – albeit not overly abundant – does support the use of multivitamins in the management of chronic stress symptoms in a variety of domains.

For example, two studies published in the same year observed a reduction in a broad array of stress symptoms after supplementation with a multi-vitamin formula for a period of only 28–30 days.

The first study (205) was a double-blind, placebo-controlled trial that involved 300 highly stressed participants. The researchers found that the participants who took a multivitamin for 30 days showed a significant reduction in stress-related symptoms, both physical and psychological.

The second study (206) was similar in design, but used a smaller sample based on more stringent exclusion criteria. Eighty participants were randomly assigned to a multivitamin or placebo group for a period of 28 days. This study also found that the group taking the multivitamin showed significant reductions in anxiety and perceived stress, as well as lower levels of fatigue and an improved ability to concentrate.

Some may argue that however high the standards of the trials were, they were short and involved a relatively small number of participants. However, when reviewing the body of literature on stress and multivitamin supplementation, the findings of these studies are repeatedly echoed.

Sara-Jane Long and David Benton from the Department of Psychology at the University of Swansea, Wales, performed one of the most comprehensive meta-analyses within this space. Long and Benton searched multiple databases for randomised, double-blind, placebo-controlled trials on the topic of stress symptoms and multivitamin supplementation (207).

In all, they identified 378 relevant studies. However, only 13 were randomised, controlled studies. Of the 13, eight fulfilled the stringent inclusion criteria. These eight studies included 1 292 healthy adult participants who took a multivitamin complex for 28–90 days. The studies assessed, amongst other things, stress, psychiatric symptoms, anxiety, depression, levels of fatigue, behaviour, and cognition.

Incredibly, in the supplementation groups, the adverse effects of stress were significantly reduced:

- perceived stress decreased by 35%
- anxiety decreased by 32%
- stress-induced psychiatric symptoms decreased by 30%, and
- self-reported levels of clarity and cognition improved by 23%.

The study came to the following conclusions:

Micronutrient supplementation has a beneficial effect on perceived stress, mild psychiatric symptoms, and aspects of everyday mood in apparently healthy individuals. Supplements containing high doses of B vitamins may be more effective in improving mood states.

There are two important conclusions we can draw from this meta-analysis:

1. High-quality multivitamins do work in chronic stress management.
2. B vitamins offer a particularly marked reduction in the adverse effects of chronic stress.

B vitamins

The role of vitamin B in stress resilience and health promotion

What is it about B vitamins that makes them so effective as mediators of the stress response?

To understand their role and importance, we have to understand a little more about their functional role in the body.

The eight B vitamins are fairly abundant in a healthy diet and can be found in a wide range of foods, including whole grains, fruits, legumes, vegetables and meats.

The most important of the B vitamins in terms of stress management and improved resilience are vitamins B6,[48] B9[49] and B12.[50] One of the primary reasons for this is that they are vital to the body's ability to produce energy. Considering that ongoing fatigue and low energy levels are common symptoms of chronic stress, this biological role is extremely valuable.

Whether instinctively, or on the recommendation of our family doctor, we often seek B-vitamin injections or supplements when we're tired, burnt out or stressed, and as the science shows, it's with good cause.

That said, arguably one of the most significant, collective roles of vitamins B6, B9 and B12 is the regulation of the amino acid,[51] homocysteine. Homocysteine is a by-product of protein metabolism that can be measured in the blood. An abnormal accumulation of homocysteine can be a marker for the development of heart disease and other major cardiovascular issues, including increased risk of heart attack, stroke, peripheral vascular disease[52] and venous blood clots. Not only does homocysteine inflict serious damage on the cardiovascular system, it also profoundly impacts the nervous system.

According to several research articles, elevated circulating homocysteine is associated with the promotion of spontaneous nerve cell death, brain shrinkage, dementia and Alzheimer's disease, and is even considered a significant risk factor for cerebrovascular disease.[53]

Here's the thing: research shows that chronic stress is associated with dramatic elevations in homocysteine (208) with potentially devastating health consequences.

This is where vitamins B12, B6 and B9 come into play. They convert homocysteine into the amino acid methionine. Whereas an elevated level of homocysteine increases the likelihood of the formation of free radicals and the resultant oxidative stress, leading to cell damage and poor health, methionine has the complete opposite effect. Methionine plays a vital role in optimal biological metabolism and several other important processes, including DNA production and repair. Remarkable to think that one of the most destructive molecules in the body has the potential to become a biologically enhancing molecule merely by the presence and actions of three B vitamins.

Even though scientists know that homocysteine has a destructive influence on the body, it is still unclear whether elevated homocysteine plays a direct and exclusive role in the disease process, or the elevation in homocysteine is merely a marker for B6, B9 and B12 deficiency.

Simply put, there is good reason to suspect that many of the health issues that accompany chronic stress are caused by vitamin B6, B9 and B12 deficiencies, which then contribute to rising levels of homocysteine.

Many studies have been published on the relationship between chronic stress and B-vitamin deficiencies. Not only does chronic stress create a greater demand for vitamins B6, B9 and B12 in the conversion of homocysteine, it also depletes all the B vitamins, most especially B6 and B12.

A study published in the *Journal of Affective Disorders* (209) identified a strong relationship between chronic stress and vitamin B6 deficiency in a group of 358 adults. The general symptoms of vitamin B6 deficiency include: fatigue, skin disorders, depression and weakened immune function. The more stress-specific symptoms are discussed later in the chapter.

In 2014, a research article by Indian researchers (210) on the topic of chronic stress, cortisol and vitamin B12 identified a mechanism by which vitamin B12 levels decline in response to chronic stress. The researchers proposed that cortisol damages particular cells in the stomach[54] that are responsible for the absorption of vitamin B12.

B-vitamin supplementation protects the brain from homocysteine-induced compromise

What we can take from the current body of scientific research is that when the body is unable to clear and metabolise homocysteine efficiently, this negatively impacts health across many domains, but most concerning are the effects on the brain, which is already a target for cortisol.

Neuro-imaging studies (211, 212) have shown that high levels of circulating homocysteine are linked to a greater incidence of brain shrinkage, as well as an elevated risk of neurological degeneration.

Remarkably, the same neuro-imaging studies show that supplementation of B-vitamins over a prolonged period of time[55] provided a certain degree of protection from brain shrinkage and neurological degenerative changes.

Not only do elevated homocysteine levels and vitamin B deficiencies result in brain atrophy and degeneration, they also result in a significant reduction in cognitive aptitude. In 2010, researchers from the Department of Pharmacology and the Department of Physiology, Anatomy and Genetics at Oxford University published a randomised control trial (212) to investigate the effects of vitamin B supplementation on homocysteine, and to determine if supplementation could slow the rate of brain atrophy and improve cognition.

The 24-month trial involved 271 subjects over the age of 70 with a history of mild cognitive impairment. Of these, 187 subjects volunteered to have cranial MRI scans[56] at the start and finish of the study. The participants were then randomly assigned to two groups of equal size. The active treatment group took vitamins B6, B9 and B12, while the other group took a placebo.

Over the two-year period, the rate of brain atrophy was 1.5% in the active treatment group and 2.16% in the placebo group. Not only was the rate of brain atrophy significantly greater in the placebo group, the researchers also noted that greater rates of brain atrophy correlated directly with lower scores on the final cognitive test. This finding of structural changes correlating with reduced and impaired cognition is by no means isolated. Numerous studies highlight this phenomenon with a high degree of reliability. Simply put, the larger your brain, the better it performs and vice versa.

The conclusion of the study is that the rate of brain shrinkage, especially in older persons, can be slowed down with treatment of the homocysteine-lowering B vitamins – B6, B9 and B12.

How do B vitamins influence general stress symptoms?

The evidence suggests that supplementation with B vitamins has a wide range of positive effects on chronic stress.

An Australian study involving 60 participants looked at the effects of 90 days of B-complex supplementation on a variety of stress outcomes (213). The high-quality, double-blind, randomised, placebo-controlled trial assessed everything from personality to work demands, mood, anxiety and even overall reported strain. While there were few to no changes in anxiety, participants taking the B-complex reported significantly lower personal strain and a reduction in cognitive and emotional compromise[57] that typically accompany chronic stress. Considering that individual differences in personality and work demands were tightly controlled, the findings provide valuable insights into the successful management of personal and organisational health and well-being.[58]

B vitamins and neurochemicals

Serotonin is a major determinant in stress resilience. Recent research is beginning to show a clear bidirectional relationship between stress and serotonin. Whereas brain serotonin reduces susceptibility to many of the adverse effects of stress, stress impairs serotonin function and possibly even production.

Researchers from the departments of Cell Biology, Neurobiology and Medicine at Duke University published an animal study (214) showing that low levels of brain serotonin lead to increased susceptibility to psychosocial stress. A reduced ability to cope with stress triggers more stress, which results in a greater degree of overall physical, mental and emotional strain.

Between 1991 and 2016, 71 high-quality molecular imaging studies showed strong evidence of stress, affective cognition and serotonin interactions. According to Margaret Davis and her team from the Department of Psychiatry at the Yale University School of Medicine (215), chronic stress may alter how serotonin acts in the brain, possibly reducing its effectiveness and predisposing those affected to a broad spectrum of psychiatric disorders.

Due to the fragility of serotonin interactions during chronic stress, it is imperative to ensure that both serotonin levels and serotonin behaviour remain optimal. Certain B vitamins, especially vitamin B6, are fundamental in the synthesis of serotonin.[59]

According to a 2016 article published in *Nutrients* (216), even the slightest vitamin B6 deficiency will result in disordered sleep, behavioural changes, impaired cardiovascular function and uncontrolled stress hormone production.

Serotonin and the microbiome

Low serotonin levels impair our ability to manage and cope with stressors, so it is imperative that we focus on positive dietary practices during periods of chronic stress. The reason is that over 90% of the body's serotonin is found in the enterochromaffin[60] cells of the digestive system. Incredibly, the synthesis of serotonin is largely influenced by the resident bacteria that reside in the digestive tract, known as the microbiome. In 2015, researchers at the California Institute of Technology (218) found that in animals with artificially compromised microbiomes, serotonin production is reduced by 60%.

In order to keep our microbiomes healthy, a diet high in fibre, protein and omega-3 fatty acids is important. Also, foods that result in intestinal stress and that cause gut inflammation, such as processed sugar, gluten and some dairy products should be kept to a minimum. Finally, only take antibiotics and cortisone-containing medications when absolutely necessary, as indiscriminate use has been shown to have devastating effects on microbiome diversity, numbers and health.

Arguably, the two most prominent B vitamins in neurochemical production are vitamins B9 and B12. The reason is that they regulate[61] the enzymes that convert amino acids both to key neurotransmitters[62] and to nitric oxide. The slightest deficiency, which is all too common in chronically stressed states, will wreak havoc with brain functioning. This deficiency could manifest in significant psychological and behavioural issues, as well as numerous metabolic disorders, such as anaemia. In fact, according to a review in *The Lancet Neurology* (217) more than a third of patients admitted to hospital for psychiatric issues have been found to have deficiencies in vitamin B9 and/or B12.

Not only do B vitamins positively influence neurological and cardiovascular health, there is some evidence that certain B vitamins, when combined with amino acids, may influence our hormonal system by increasing growth hormone output.

As previously mentioned, growth hormone is responsible for numerous biological functions including cell reproduction and growth, DNA integrity, strong bones, youthful skin, neurological integrity, muscle tone, muscle size, and optimal functioning of the cardiovascular and immune systems. Protracted elevations of cortisol and adrenalin have been shown to lower several hormones that ensure physical integrity, including growth hormone and testosterone (in men). This change in hormone profile may contribute to the weakened physical state commonly associated with chronic stress. While vitamin B supplementation may seem promising, a lot more research needs to be done in this space before clear conclusions can be drawn.

Despite the important role of B vitamins in a variety of important biological settings, levels appear to be highly unstable in industrialised nations. There are numerous reasons for this, but it is safe to say that the major factors promoting deficiencies are stress, specific genetic polymorphisms,[63] gender, ethnicity, hormonal dysfunction, regular use of medications, drugs, alcohol, poor diet, obesity, poor exercise behaviours, and advancing age.

Vitamin B6, B9 and B12 deficiencies are becoming increasingly widespread. United Kingdom government statistics from national diet and nutrition surveys (219) show that 3–5% of the adult population are B9 and B12 deficient. The same survey found that lower socio-economic groups show rates of vitamin B9 and B12 deficiencies that are twice as high as those of more advantaged communities. The reason may be higher levels of stress and limited access to nutrient-rich foods, which are expensive.

The US statistics are even more alarming. According to the Centers for Disease Control (220), 10.5% of the entire US population are deficient in vitamin B6. Considering the role of vitamin B6 in stress hormone regulation and neurochemical balance, this could have profound effects in terms of dysregulation of the stress response.

Advancing age is a major factor in the development of vitamin B deficiencies. As we age, both our absorption and metabolism of B vitamins becomes significantly less effective. Combined with a lifetime of compounded stress, this can contribute to nutrient deficiencies at a stage in our lives when we can least afford it.

According to a 2007 article published in *The American Journal of Clinical Nutrition* (221), 30% of adults over the age of 60 have significant deficiencies of vitamin B12. Vitamin B1[64] deficiency is also common in older populations. According to New Zealand researchers (222), the prevalence of vitamin B1 deficiencies may be as high as 16 to 18% in older populations. Not only are vitamin B1, B6, B9 and B12 deficiencies becoming increasingly more prevalent across all populations, so are deficiencies in vitamin B2. What makes this so concerning is that vitamin B2 influences countless cellular processes including the synthesis, conversion and recycling of vitamins B3, B9 and B12. This functional interplay is important in stress management and resilience.

Vitamin B2 deficiency is exceptionally common. According to the *Handbook of Behavior, Food and Nutrition* (223) vitamin B2 deficiency affects 10% to 15% of the world's population.

Multivitamin supplementation

Multivitamins are an over-the-counter nutritional supplement that typically contain both water-soluble and lipid-soluble vitamins together with a range of essential minerals. According to an article published in *The American Journal of Clinical Nutrition* (224), multivitamin supplementation is a practice that dates back to the 1940s. Despite the lucrative market and growing demand, it is concerning that there is currently no standard or regulatory definition for nutritional products of this nature (225). Due to the lack of regulation and standardisation, product compositions are highly variable in terms of nutrients, quantities and, most concerning, quality.

Safety of multivitamin supplements

According to the National Institutes of Health (226), most of the once-daily multivitamin supplements contain all or most of the more recognised vitamins and minerals, generally at levels close to the Daily Values (DVs), Recommended Dietary Allowance (RDAs) or Adequate Intakes (AIs) for these nutrients. However, formulations for children, adults, men, women, pregnant women and seniors typically provide varied amounts of the same vitamins based on the perceived needs of these populations.

This doesn't mean that none of the multivitamin supplements contain significantly higher RDA levels of certain nutrients. There are products in the marketplace that contain nutritional profiles that well exceed accepted safety limits with little consideration for the long-term implications on health outcomes (227). Another common practice is the incorporation of a wide variety of herbal ingredients, some of which have medicinal properties and strong biological influences.

Multivitamin supplements should not be confused with specialised nutraceuticals, such as those taken with a specific intention. For example, dietary supplements may be used for enhanced physical performance, improved energy, weight control, improved immune regulation or the management of specific health issues. In these instances, nutrients often exceed conservative dietary guidelines.

> **Warning:** Do not take dietary supplements without consulting a trained professional. This applies to all the supplements covered in this section.

According to the National Institutes of Health (228), taking a basic multivitamin supplement that provides nutrients close to conservative recommended intakes should pose no safety risks to healthy people. However, those who take multiple nutritional supplements and/or who eat fortified foods and beverages should be aware that the combination may elevate nutrient intakes beyond the upper limits and increase the risk of adverse health effects. For this reason, consult a health professional for guidance and advice rather than the enthusiastic salesperson at the retail store.

There are certain sub-groups within the broader population who need to exercise far more caution when it comes to multivitamin supplementation. This group will include smokers and pregnant women, especially with overconsumption of vitamin A.[65] Additionally, men and children should be careful of excess supplementary iron. As a general rule, men shouldn't exceed their recommended dietary allowance of 8 mg per day. Children run the risk of severe poisoning from excess iron. According to a report by the American Association of Poison Control Centers (229), supplements containing iron are a leading cause of poisoning in children under the age of six.

Interactions with medications

Multivitamin supplements that provide nutrients at recommended intake levels do not ordinarily interact with medications. However, there is one important exception. The National Institutes of Health (228) advise those who take medications to reduce blood clotting to be cautious about any dietary supplement that contains vitamin K. Vitamin K may interfere with the effectiveness of these medications.

Choosing the best product

When choosing a multivitamin supplement, always opt for a reputable brand with a large international market presence. Certificates of quality and authenticity are important, as is regular third-party testing. You should select a product that is tailored to your age, gender or other potentially unique characteristics, such as pregnancy and sports activities.

B-vitamin supplementation

Dosage and safe limits

The B vitamins are water-soluble: any excess is generally excreted in urine, so they are typically safe at doses much higher than standardised guidelines (RDAs). However, their water-solubility also means that they require a more consistent consumption. According to an analysis entitled "B Vitamins and the brain: mechanisms, dose and efficacy – a review" (230) only three of the eight B vitamins have been ascribed any upper limit for daily consumption – B3, B6 and B9. The others are considered fairly safe irrespective of dose.

These upper limits must be taken seriously because the negative health implications are severe, as you'll learn later in this chapter.

Vitamin B6 (pyridoxine)

Vitamin B6 is the first of the three B vitamins with a suggested upper limit. According to the US Food and Nutrition Board (231), the RDA for vitamin B6 will vary slightly depending on age and gender:

- teenagers should consume around 1 mg per day
- adults between the ages of 18 and 50 should have around 1.3 mg per day, and
- over 50s require somewhat higher intakes, ranging from 1.5 mg for women to 1.7 mg for men per day.

As you know, when it comes to nutrient supplementation, *less is always more*! Higher doses of many vitamins and minerals over prolonged periods of time can be not only ineffectual, but also detrimental to health. For example, several studies show that chronic administration of high doses (1–6 g per day) of vitamin B6 for a period of 12 to 40 months can cause significant neurological issues. Symptoms may include loss of control over bodily movements. The severity of neurological compromise in response to an overdose will usually cease when vitamin B6 supplementation is discontinued.

The bioavailability of vitamin B6, whether from supplements[66] or natural food sources, is in the region of 75% (231). Although absorption rates are higher than many other vitamins and minerals, we must consider that excretion is very rapid. This explains the need for steady but moderate intake.

While over-dosage frequently occurs with dietary supplements, no over-dosage has ever been reported from food sources. The richest and most bioavailable dietary sources of vitamin B6 include fish, beef liver and other organ meats, potatoes, starchy vegetables, and all fruits except citrus.

Consider that certain health issues and medications can create abnormally low vitamin B6 levels. People suffering from digestive health disorders such as celiac disease, Crohn's disease and ulcerative colitis are often deficient in vitamin B6. Anti-seizure medications, asthma medications and medications used to treat rheumatoid arthritis are associated with changes in vitamin B6 status.

Vitamin B9 (folate)

Vitamin B9 is the second of the three B vitamins with a suggested upper limit. Like vitamin B6, vitamin B9 cannot be consumed in excess without health implications. According to the US Food and Nutrition Board (231), the RDA for vitamin B9 will vary slightly depending on age, but not necessarily gender:

- the suggested intake for persons under 13 is 200–300 mcg[67] per day
- for persons aged 14 and older, the RDA is 400 mcg per day
- the RDA during pregnancy and lactation is somewhat higher, ranging from 500–600 mcg per day, and
- the upper limit of vitamin B9 supplementation in persons over 19 is 1 000 mcg per day, beyond which health risks may increase.

According to the National Institutes of Health (228), about 85% of supplemental vitamin B9 is bioavailable when taken with food. Interestingly, when consumed without food, nearly 100% of the vitamin is bioavailable. This suggests that supplementing on an empty stomach may be the most effective means of maintaining vitamin B9 status, and potentially other micronutrients[68] as well.

At high doses, vitamin B9 does not necessarily create toxicity – although there are suggestions of impaired immune functioning – but it can exacerbate the damage done by an insufficiency of vitamin B12,[69] especially in terms of cognition (232). Simply put, if you have an existing vitamin B12 deficiency, the negative health associations attributed to this deficit will be profoundly amplified when supplementing with *excess* vitamin B9.

Extremely high vitamin B9 intake may result in negative interactions with a variety of medications, such as those prescribed for rheumatoid arthritis, psoriasis, cancer, infections and even malaria.

Several medications and practices can create severe vitamin B9 deficiencies through reduced absorption, increased excretion, or both. These include chronic alcohol consumption, antacids, H2 blockers,[70] non-steroidal anti-inflammatories (ibuprofen), anti-seizure and some immune-modulating medications. Additionally, persons who suffer from digestive conditions such as ulcerative colitis, celiac and Crohn's disease, or who have had gastric surgery, are more prone to vitamin B9 deficiency.

Vitamin B9 is easily obtained through proper dietary practices as it is found in a wide variety of foods, including vegetables – especially dark-green, leafy vegetables – fruits, nuts, legumes, dairy products, poultry and meat, eggs, seafood and grains. The foods that are the richest source of B9 include spinach, liver, yeast, asparagus and Brussels sprouts.

Vitamin B3 (niacin)

Vitamin B3 is the third of the three B vitamins with a suggested upper limit. The recommended daily dietary allowance for vitamin B3 varies slightly depending on age and gender. On the whole, the intake guidelines for females are slightly lower than males in all age groups:

- persons under 18 require 8–16 mg per day
- women over 18 require 14 mg per day, whereas men require 16 mg per day
- the safe upper limit for vitamin B3 consumption is in the region of 35 mg per day.

High doses of 50 mg and more can be associated with numerous side effects. The most common side effect is known as 'niacin flush', which is best described as a burning, tingling sensation in the face and chest area together with red or flushed skin. According to the *American Journal of Cardiovascular Drugs* (233), taking an aspirin 30 minutes prior to the vitamin B3 may help reduce these symptoms. This practice would only be necessary if severe deficiencies and sensitivities coexist.

It is important to consider that very high doses[71] may result in liver damage and stomach ulcers. If you have been prescribed high doses, make sure your doctor regularly tests your liver function. Medical experts warn that persons with a history of liver disease, kidney disease and/or stomach ulcers should be very cautious about taking vitamin B3 supplements. Excessive consumption can exacerbate allergies,[72] lower blood pressure, provoke certain autoimmune conditions, and possibly raise the risk of heart rhythm disorders.

There are several medications that have strong interactions with vitamin B3, either by reducing effectiveness or by promoting vitamin B3 deficiency. Some of these include antibiotics,[73] anti-seizure medications, blood pressure medications, alpha-blockers, cholesterol-lowering medications, and certain diabetic medications.

Foods high in vitamin B3 are not associated with overdose side effects. The best sources include fish, poultry, meat, organ meat, some legumes, and vegetables (broccoli, beetroot, asparagus).

General supplementation guidelines

According to a 2016 review in *Nutrients* (230), the other B vitamins (B1, B2,

B5, B7 and B12) can generally be consumed in amounts many times the RDA without any adverse effects. However, serious concerns have been raised over high doses of isolated B vitamins and health outcomes.

Why choose a multivitamin or B-complex over isolates?

There have been several reports in recent years suggesting links between excessive vitamin B supplementation and an increased incidence of cancers. In 2009, a large research team from the Department of Heart Disease at the Haukeland University Hospital in Norway published a study on the long-term associations of B-vitamin supplementation,[74] cancer prevalence and all-cause mortality (234).

The analysis included two randomised, double-blind, placebo-controlled clinical trials[75] involving a total of 6 837 participants with ischaemic heart disease. The patients were treated with varying combinations of B vitamins or a placebo and were then monitored for nine years. The various supplementation protocols that were used included a combination of vitamin B6, B9 and B12; a combination of B9 and B12; vitamin B6 in isolation, and a placebo.

Disturbingly, the data revealed that the combination of high-dose B9 and B12 increased the risk of developing cancer by 21% and was also associated with a marked increase in mortality from all causes. Oddly enough, of the supplementation groups, only the group taking vitamin B6 in isolation appeared to be unaffected. However, other studies show very different outcomes pertaining to isolated vitamin B6 intake.

Because of the high prevalence of supplemental vitamin B use, any possible increased association with disease warrants extensive investigation.

A group of researchers from multiple institutions set out to probe this asso-ciation in the most detailed study of its kind (235). The primary focus was to assess the ten-year relationship between lung cancer[76] risk and the average daily consumption of individual B-vitamin as well as multivitamin supplementation.

A total of 77 118 participants aged 50 to 76 years were recruited over a two-year period. To ensure reliable findings, numerous factors were considered that included smoking, race, age, education, body size, personal history of cancer or chronic lung disease, alcohol consumption, family history of lung cancer, and use of anti-inflammatory drugs.

The results were alarming. While women appeared to be unaffected by supplemental use of vitamins B6, B9 and B12, men showed extremely strong cancer associations. The use of vitamins B6 and B12 from individual supplement sources was associated with a 30 to 40% increase in lung cancer risk.

When the ten-year average supplement dose was evaluated, there was an almost 200% increase in lung cancer risk among men in the highest categories of vitamin B6 (>20 mg per day) and B12 (>55µg per day) compared with non-users.[77] The combination of smoking and excessive B6 and B12 intake was by far the greatest risk group.

Interestingly, when B vitamins were consumed as part of multivitamin supplements, there was no additional disease risk in either men or women. The mechanisms underlying this finding remain unclear.

More research is necessary before definitive guidelines can be established. However, we have to consider the benefits of B-vitamin supplementation in the context of chronic stress and health outcomes and weigh those benefits against the risks. Mitigating the risks is possible by taking low supplement doses and by selecting multivitamins or more comprehensive B-complex formulations rather than isolated nutrients.

Adaptogens – a force to be reckoned with

Adaptogens are nothing short of a secret weapon we can use to combat chronic stress. They are a group of plant-derived compounds that are known to increase attention and endurance when in a state of fatigue. They are also able to significantly reduce stress-induced impairments and disorders related to multiple systems, including the nervous, hormonal, cardiovascular and immune systems.

For more than 60 years, adaptogens have been studied and thoroughly investigated in relation to physiology, pharmacology, toxicology and potential uses in medicine and the management of stress-related health disorders.

Adaptogens are unique in the way that they enable the body to successfully adapt to numerous environmental factors – both external and internal – thereby preventing subsequent or potential damage. Simply put, they are master metabolic regulators.

Many of the more common adaptogenic plants have been used in traditional Chinese medicine and Ayurveda[78] for centuries, before the advent of modern-day stress, to promote physical and mental health, improve the body's defence mechanisms, and enhance longevity.

What's remarkable about adaptogens is that the normal paradigm of a single medication for a single disease does not apply because adaptogens can have multiple, sometimes overlapping, pharmacological and biological effects. The reason is that they exhibit multi-target action and interact with a number of cellular receptors[79] (236). Simply put, they interface with and influence many different types of cells.

Of particular relevance in the successful management of chronic stress and the promotion of stress resilience is that adaptogens are able to strongly influence the body's response to numerous neurochemicals and hormones, especially stress hormones, steroid hormones and even serotonin.

According to a 2017 literature review published in the *Annals of the New York Academy of Sciences* (237):

A characteristic feature of adaptogens is that they act as eustressors (i.e., "good stressors") and as mild stress mimetics or "stress vaccines" that induce stress-protective responses.

Within the body and broader cellular machinery, mild stress induced by adaptogens promotes a resistance or 'immunity' to more severe or protracted stress exposure. However, there is a drawback in that this resistance carries no memory function. This means that regular repeated exposure to adaptogenic compounds would be required in order to maintain a stress-resistant state.

The best example of this model is physical exercise. Physical exercise is a form of mild, short-lived stress that is usually progressive in nature. Regular exposure increases resilience to the activity and over time enhances our capacities in that area – aerobic, strength, speed, flexibility. When we stop exercising, our ability to withstand the same physical stressors diminishes progressively over a relatively short period of time.

An important note on healthy stress (eustress)

To fully appreciate the potential that adaptogens offer in an overall stress resilience model, you have to understand that from a biological perspective, there are positive stressors (eustressors) and negative stressors. Fundamentally, a eustressor challenges the body, but does not overwhelm it. This manageable challenge then strengthens, up-regulates and enhances numerous biological systems so that the next time the body is confronted with a similar challenge, the relative demands are lessened and the threat averted.

Eustress creates a manageable challenge to our cellular machinery giving it the opportunity for considerable up-regulation of all the working components. A good example of this effect can be observed in the brain when exposed to three eustress environments: cognitive challenges (learning and memory), sporadic dietary restriction (intermittent fasting) and physical exercise.

The eustressor triggers the release of several neurochemicals including serotonin, glutamate and acetylcholine. These neurotransmitters enhance attention, memory, motivation, arousal, cognition and learning. Not only does the increased activity of these neurochemicals enhance and improve brain functionality, they also trigger several chemical processes within the brain cells themselves, which promotes their structural integrity. These include:

- an increase in BDNF
- enhanced DNA repair
- the expression of proteins[90] that protect the structure of the cells
- the activation of antioxidant enzymes, and
- up-regulation of anti-carcinogenic and anti-ageing proteins.[81]

The overall effect is vastly improved structure, integrity and functionality of the brain. Conversely, should the cognitive/emotional challenge become too great, food intake become restricted for too long, or physical exercise become too demanding, the eustressor becomes a negative stressor, which would then result in systemic breakdown instead of enhancement.

Like regular physical exercise, repeated administration of adaptogens and the subsequent stress-protective responses invariably leads to prolonged general resistance in multiple domains, specifically in mental and physical endurance.

The role of adaptogens in moderating stress and promoting resilience is multifactorial and complex. Interestingly, adaptogens influence both the stress axis (HPA) and our cells.

While adaptogenic plants are able to reduce cortisol and stress hormone responses to stressors, as well as enhance and expedite the normalisation of biological functioning following one of life's many challenges, the primary value of adaptogens lies in their direct influence on our cells.

Typically, stress triggers the formation of chemicals[82] and proteins[83] that promote cellular damage[84] and suppress the production of energy in the cell.

This reduced energy production in our cells is especially destructive because several proteins, such as Hsp70, rely on this valuable energy to perform ongoing cell repair and maintenance. The impact of this down-regulation may result in cell damage, abnormalities or even premature death. Additionally, stress can trigger intrinsic proteins[85] that corrupt the cell's responsiveness and interaction with cortisol.

According to a 2010 review published in *Pharmaceuticals* (238), many of the commonly used adaptogens positively influence our cells' relationship to cortisol, reduce free radical production, and are able to increase energy production as well as facilitate enhanced repair of damaged proteins.

There are over 70 adaptogenic plants, some of which have been extensively researched. The more commonly used adaptogens include ashwagandha, *Bacopa monnieri*, *Rhodiola rosea*, *Cordyceps sinensis*, licorice, *Schisandra chinensis*, holy basil, *Polygala tenuifolia*, *Rehmannia glutinosa*, Asian ginseng, and the better-known Siberian ginseng.

Intriguingly, each adaptogen has completely unique characteristics, inducing an extensive range of biological effects, many of which are only now being uncovered. I've chosen to discuss three very different adaptogens to illustrate the diversity of their effects:

- *Rhodiola rosea*
- Ashwagandha (*Withania somnifera*)
- *Bacopa monnieri*.

Rhodiola rosea

The *Rhodiola rosea* plant, also known as arctic root, is typically found at high altitudes of 1 000–5 000 metres above sea level in the northern latitudes. Researchers from the Swedish Herbal Institute and the University of Melbourne have identified over 140 chemical compounds in this unique health-promoting herb (239). Due to its purported adaptogenic properties, it has been studied for its performance-enhancing capabilities in healthy populations as well as its therapeutic properties in a number of clinical populations.

In 2015, a randomised, controlled trial (240) on the efficacy of adaptogenic supplements for stress resilience, assessed the impact of *Rhodiola rosea*, *Schisandra chinensis* and Siberian ginseng on physical and emotional stress-induced loss of concentration, coordination, fatigue and hormonal balance in 215 elite athletes between the ages of 18 and 35. One group received adaptogenic supplements, the other group received a placebo.

A broad array of tests, including psychological, neurological and hormonal, were performed at the beginning of the study, and again after 7, 8, 28 and 29 days of daily oral administration. Fatigue was chosen as one of the primary indicators and was measured using multiple rating systems.

Additionally, blood testosterone-to-cortisol ratios, as well as lactic acid, were assessed to gauge recovery from intense training and competition. The study found significant differences between the placebo and adaptogen groups in all domains, including reported fatigue, perceived stress, attention/focus, hormonal balance, physical tests and sporting performance.

The researchers concluded that supplementation with adaptogenic preparations, including *Rhodiola rosea*, increases physical performance and the recovery of athletes after heavy physical and emotional loads. The authors believe that because adaptogens enhance the body's ability to withstand physical and emotional stress, these compounds may be useful in the recovery process following exercise and in the prevention of the symptoms of overtraining.

Another remarkable discovery was published in *Frontiers in Nutrition* in 2015 (241). A team of researchers from several universities collaborated to investigate the antiviral properties of *Rhodiola rosea*. The study followed 48 marathon runners, randomly divided into two equal groups. One group of runners (6 females and 18 males) ingested 600 mg of *Rhodiola rosea* per day, while the other group (7 females and 17 males) received a placebo for 30 days prior to the marathon and 7 days after the marathon.

It is established that during prolonged strenuous exercise, there is a substantial increase in free radical production resulting in cell compromise, structural damage to muscle fibre ultrastructure,[86] increased systemic inflammation and transient immune dysfunction (242). This temporary compromise to the immune system is associated with an increased incidence and severity of acute respiratory infections. If you exercise vigorously on a regular basis, you'll know this all too well.

The study showed that the group supplementing with *Rhodiola rosea* had a lower risk of developing viral infections following prolonged, intense endurance exercise. The reason appears to be related to bioactive compounds that induce robust, antiviral activity.

According to the authors:

> *Our results indicate that* Rhodiola rosea *supplementation has the potential to protect athletes from exercise-induced susceptibility to infections by attenuating virus replication.*

These findings are especially relevant in the context of chronic stress, since prolonged cortisol elevation results in increased susceptibility to colds and flu. Therefore, any natural, non-toxic substance or compound that has antiviral properties is invaluable in terms of stress resilience.

In 2009, Erik Olsson of the Department of Psychology at Uppsala University in Sweden published a study on the effectiveness of *Rhodiola rosea* in the management of stress-related fatigue (243). The study was a randomised, double-blind, placebo-controlled trial involving 60 participants between the ages of 20 and 55.

They were randomised into two equal-sized groups: one group received 576 mg of *Rhodiola rosea* extract per day, while the other group received a placebo. Quality of life, symptoms of fatigue, depression, attention and salivary cortisol (in the morning) were assessed on the first day and after 28 days of supplementation.

Comparison between the two groups found that the participants who took the *Rhodiola rosea* extract experienced less burnout and their cortisol levels were considerably lower.

The study suggests that repeated administration of *Rhodiola rosea* exerts an anti-fatigue effect that increases mental performance, particularly the ability to concentrate, and decreases cortisol in burnout patients with chronic fatigue syndrome.

This study was the first to demonstrate clinically that *Rhodiola rosea* exerts its beneficial health effects on stress-induced disorders through modulation of the most important stress marker, cortisol.

In 2012, a European trial was published in *Phytotherapy Research* that investigated the therapeutic effects and safety of four weeks of treatment with *Rhodiola rosea* in subjects suffering from chronic stress and associated health symptoms (244). The trial involved 101 participants who received a dose of 200 mg of *Rhodiola rosea* twice daily for a period of four weeks. Extensive assessments covering various aspects of stress symptoms and adverse events were incorporated into the study.

Invariably, all tests showed clinically relevant improvements in stress symptoms, disability, functional impairment and overall therapeutic effect. Remarkably, improvements were observed within just three days of treatment and continued for the rest of the trial.

The authors concluded by saying that 200 mg of *Rhodiola rosea* twice a day[87] for four weeks is safe and effective in improving life-stress symptoms to a clinically relevant degree.

While *Rhodiola rosea* contains numerous bioactive compounds, one of the most impactful appears to be salidroside. Research has shown (238) that salidroside has strong neuroprotective activity, which reduces the risk of stress-induced conditions, and disorders related to the nervous, hormonal and immune systems. In 2008, Chinese researchers published a study in *Cellular and Molecular Neurobiology* suggesting that salidroside may be effective in treating and preventing strokes and neurodegenerative diseases such as Alzheimer's and Parkinson's (245).

Not only does the literature indicate that *Rhodiola rosea* has a protective influence in the context of the brain and circulatory system, it also appears that this arctic plant may enhance their functionality as well. In 2009, Swiss researchers (246) identified yet another unique compound contained within *Rhodiola rosea*. This composite (monoterpene glucoside rosiridin) has been found to inhibit and slow down the removal of neurochemicals in the brain. This is especially significant when we consider that this effect may promote greater functionality in both the cognitive and emotional spaces. In fact, this is the mechanism by which many commonly prescribed behavioural and attention-promoting medications operate. Knowing that chronic stress negatively impacts numerous neurochemicals, including serotonin, this effect could be highly advantageous in maintaining behavioural and cognitive integrity during times of ongoing crisis.

Concerns

While typical concerns with botanicals, nutraceuticals and pharmaceuticals revolve around side effects and long-term health associations, the current body of evidence indicates that there are few to no clinically significant side effects (247) when taking *Rhodiola rosea*. However, there are two issues to be aware of. The first is the methodological quality of many of the studies and the second is the quality of the preparations that are currently commercially available.

There have been hundreds of studies in multiple languages that support the effectiveness of *Rhodiola rosea* in a variety of health domains, including stress protection, cardiovascular protection, anti-ageing, enhanced cognition, and hormonal stabilisation. However, many are considered weak by the experts. Furthermore, there are only a dozen randomised, controlled trials, some of which are included in our discussion. However, only about six studies rate high on the Oxford scoring system for methodological quality. However promising the findings seem, bear in mind that more research may be required to validate the existing data and to provide exact dose prescriptions.

Current dosage guidelines

Acute use for the management of fatigue and chronic stress	288–680 mg per day
Daily prevention against fatigue	50 mg per day
Safety limits	680 mg per day

Again, the dubious quality and authenticity of available products is a major concern. In 2016, researchers from the UK, Germany, China and Switzerland published a study (248) in which 40 commercial products[88] sourced from different suppliers were analysed.

The findings showed that consistency of the products varied significantly. Approximately 20% of commercial products that claimed to be *Rhodiola rosea* did not contain a principal constituent known as rosavin, which distinguishes *Rhodiola rosea* from other closely related plant species. In fact, these manufacturers were using cheaper, closely related plants. Moreover, some of these products appeared not to contain salidroside, yet another marker compound found in *Rhodiola rosea* and in no other species.

Approximately 80% of the remaining commercial products were lower in rosavin content than registered medicinal products, and also appeared to be adulterated with other plant species.

All in all, the same principles that apply to vitamins apply here. Choose products from reputable companies with a long-standing reputation in the industry. Certificates of authenticity and third-party testing may also be beneficial.

Ashwagandha

Ashwagandha, also known as *Withania somnifera* or Indian ginseng, is a herb that has been extensively used in Ayurvedic medicine for thousands of years. This unique plant from the nightshade family[89] is one of the most widely researched adaptogens. It has been studied in relation to its antioxidant, anti-carcinogenic, anti-anxiety, antidepressant, cardio-protective, thyroid modulating, immune-modulating, anti-bacterial, anti-fungal, anti-inflammatory, neuroprotective and cognitive-enhancing effects.

Over 35 chemical constituents have been isolated from ashwagandha that have been shown to protect cells from oxidative damage and disease in a variety of research settings.

In 2012, the *Indian Journal of Psychological Medicine* published a study on the effectiveness of ashwagandha in buffering the adverse effects of stress in adults (249).

The study was a prospective, double-blind, randomised, placebo-controlled trial involving a total of 64 subjects with an ongoing history of chronic stress. Prior to the study, extensive evaluations were performed on the participants, which encompassed physiological markers, such as cortisol levels, as well as an exhaustive series of psychological assessments.

Following this initial evaluation, participants were randomised to either a placebo group or a treatment group (300 mg), who were instructed to take one capsule twice a day for a period of 60 days. To ensure compliance, and to assess whether or not the participants experienced adverse reactions, the research team performed regular follow-ups on both groups. The final safety and efficacy assessments were done on day 60 of the trial.

Remarkably, the treatment group showed a 44% reduction in perceived stress, whereas the placebo group reported only a 5.5% reduction. Additionally, at the end of the trial, the treatment group showed a 27.9% drop in blood cortisol levels, compared with only 7.9% in the placebo group. Neither the treatment nor placebo groups reported any significant side effects.

The authors concluded:

> *The findings of this study suggest that a high-concentration, full-spectrum ashwagandha root extract safely and effectively improves an individual's resistance towards stress and thereby improves self-assessed quality of life.*

This was by no means an isolated study. Similar findings were published in 2017 in the *Journal of Evidence-Based Complementary and Alternative Medicine* (250). Not only did the more recent study assess the psychological and physiological stress-buffering effects of ashwagandha, but also the influence that the plant has on eating behaviours and weight control during periods of chronic stress.

In this study on the relationship between ashwagandha supplementation and weight during periods of chronic stress, 52 subjects were randomly assigned to a placebo group or treatment group receiving 600 mg of ashwagandha root extract per day for a period of eight weeks.

Initial evaluations revealed that all subjects were experiencing chronic stress and a plethora of adverse effects. Their symptoms included, but were not limited to, concentration issues, insomnia, anxiety, restlessness, physical exhaustion, mental fatigue and headaches.

Interestingly, the study showed that both groups showed a reduction in stress symptoms during various intervals of the trial. However, the treatment group reported a 33% reduction in stress symptoms! In fact, the treatment group showed a considerably higher degree of improvement across all cognitive and emotional domains. But the most impactful outcomes of the study related to weight and cortisol levels.

Both the treatment and placebo groups had similar serum cortisol levels at the start of the trial. However, by the eighth week, the overall blood cortisol levels of the treatment group dropped by around 22%.

Moreover, overall body weight for both groups dropped during the period of the study. However, the treatment group lost at least twice as much weight as the placebo group. Remarkably, those supplementing with ashwagandha lost more than 3% of their body weight.

The authors concluded:

The results of this study suggest that ashwagandha root extract reduces psychological and physiological markers of stress, improves mental well-being, and reduces serum (blood) cortisol level and food cravings, and improves eating behaviours. A statistically significant reduction in body weight and body mass index were observed in patients treated with ashwagandha root extract compared to placebo. Therefore, we conclude that ashwagandha root extract can be useful for body-weight management in patients experiencing chronic stress.

Other benefits of ashwagandha supplementation during periods of chronic stress include improved sleep, neuroprotection and even enhanced cognition.

There have been several animal studies investigating the mechanistic influence of ashwagandha in terms of protecting the brain and nervous system. Seeing that chronic stress results in compositional changes, disruptions in connectivity and even reductions in brain mass, this could be a significant advantage associated with ashwagandha supplementation.

It has been well established in the literature that ashwagandha up-regulates antioxidant enzymes in the brain, thereby protecting it from free radical damage. However, there appears to be far more to its role of protecting the brain from stress-induced disorders. In 2009, *Neurochemical Research* published an animal study investigating the neuroprotective role of *Withania somnifera*[90] (251).

Following the study the authors concluded:

> *These observations thus suggest that WS root extract could be developed as a potential preventive or therapeutic drug for stress-induced neurological disorders.*

These comments stem from findings that ashwagandha has been shown not only to up-regulate antioxidant enzymes, but also to suppress both excessive nitric oxide and stress hormone release, in addition to increasing the serotonin levels within certain key regions of the brain.

There has been growing interest in recent years about the possible therapeutic applications of *Withania somnifera* in the prevention and treatment of neurodegenerative diseases including Alzheimer's, Huntington's, Parkinson's and spinal cord injuries. In 2014, Japanese researchers performed an in-depth investigation into ashwagandha's effect on certain neurodegenerative disorders (252). This particular study focused on spinal cord injuries and Alzheimer's disease. One of the stand-out features of this study was the fact that it showed that various constituents of ashwagandha can actually combat Alzheimer's and even facilitate dramatic nerve regeneration.

The study also draws on extensive research showing that in Alzheimer's disease models and dementia, ashwagandha extract can functionally promote nerve growth, enhance memory, protect brain cells and promote the clearance of amyloid plaques.[91] Not only has ashwagandha been shown to influence Alzheimer's and dementia, but also Parkinson's and Huntington's by means of promoting functional recovery through up-regulation of antioxidant pathways, in addition to exerting a neuroprotective effect (253, 254).

Ashwagandha may even be effective in improving sleep quality during periods of stress. Although human research is still limited, numerous animal models showing the effectiveness of *Withania somnifera* in sleep promotion have been published over the years. Two animal studies by a team of researchers from the University Institute of Pharmaceutical Science at Panjab University in India (255, 256) found that high doses of ashwagandha (100–200 mg per kilogram) had the same effects on sleep latency and quality as the commonly prescribed tranquilliser diazepam. The mechanism by which ashwagandha is thought to affect sleep is through up-regulation in the activity of an important neurochemical found in the brain called gamma-Aminobutyric acid (GABA). This neurotransmitter reduces overexcitability of nerve cells, promoting a sense of calm, and is essential in maintaining optimal biological balance.

Current dosage guidelines

The lowest effective dose for infrequent usage	300–500 mg per day
Optimal dose	6000 mg per day (divided into 3 doses)
Lowest dosage for chronic use	50–100 mg per day

It should be noted that ashwagandha root extract is the preferred form of ashwagandha for the purposes of supplementation. Also, ashwagandha is best taken with meals. If you plan on supplementing once a day, breakfast is the recommended meal.

The current body of literature reports a low level of toxicity in ashwagandha, even at extremely high doses. Interestingly, the herb acts synergistically with numerous medications and even alcohol. Even so, exercise caution when combining ashwagandha with first-generation antidepressants, specifically monoamine oxidase (MAO) inhibitors. This is not surprising seeing that many nutrients and medications have negative interactions with MAO inhibitors, which is one of the reasons that this class of medication has been replaced with newer generation options.

Bacopa monnieri

Bacopa monnieri – commonly known as water hyssop or Brahmi – has also been used in traditional Ayurvedic medicine for thousands of years. *Bacopa monnieri* has exceptionally strong adaptogenic properties and is typically prescribed for anxiety, depression, learning disorders, memory decline, inflammation, pain, fevers, blood disorders, and even heavy-metal poisoning.

Although *Bacopa monnieri* exerts a direct influence on the stress axis, this adaptogen may be most effective when used as part of a rebuilding model during or after periods of chronic stress, specifically in enhancing cognition and stabilising mood.

Bacopa monnieri combats stress-induced compromise of memory and learning ability

In 2010, Australian researchers published a study investigating the effectiveness of _Bacopa monnieri_ on the improvement of memory in older persons (257). The three-month study was a randomised, double-blind, placebo-controlled trial involving 98 healthy participants over the age of 55.

Participants were randomised into two groups, one of which received _Bacopa monnieri_ at a dose of 300 mg per day and the other an identical placebo. Neuropsychological and subjective memory assessments were performed at the beginning and at the end of the trial.

The results of the three-month study found that those supplementing with _Bacopa monnieri_ showed considerable improvements in working memory and learning ability when compared with the placebo group.

This biological effect associated with _Bacopa monnieri_ supplementation is significant in the framework of chronic stress, as cognitive decline is a common comorbidity.[92] According to a research article published in _Neurobiology of Learning and Memory_ (258) exposure to both acute and chronic stress has a detrimental effect on working memory as well as learning ability, for several reasons. This said, the primary mechanism underlying the down-regulation of cognitive functionality in response to stress exposure is believed to be attributed to reduced BDNF production and signalling.[93]

At some point in our lives, we have all experienced stress-associated memory compromise. Stress-induced recall failure can occur gradually or rapidly at any point along the stress continuum.

I have to confess that one of my more embarrassing moments in life had to do with high levels of stress, correspondingly elevated cortisol, and sudden memory loss.

SEVERAL YEARS AGO I MET the most striking woman. Exceedingly attractive, highly intelligent, stylish, charismatic, not to mention kind and generous – she was nothing short of perfect, and still is. The electricity and chemistry between us was intoxicating. Overwhelmed by our interpersonal dynamic, I didn't seize the opportunity to ask her out.

A few weeks passed, but it felt like years. She was constantly on my mind. During this time I couldn't concentrate on work, couldn't sleep and even briefly lost my appetite. The lack of sleep spiked my cortisol, creating chaos and disruption within all my major systems. It got to the point where I could not continue to live in this disorganised state – it was time to act. Finally, I did. In a moment of bravery – or desperation to normalise my overexcited state – I asked her if she wanted to meet. At the time, my stress axis was in complete overdrive, to the extent that I was shaking like a leaf. I certainly wasn't 18 – more like 40 – and this was not the first date I had been on. Yet I couldn't gather myself, let alone remain centred. She enthusiastically agreed and later that day we found ourselves drinking herbal tea in a quiet garden setting.

There I was, perfectly positioned to entice her, perhaps even impress her, but for some reason my mouth and brain had a major disconnect. Odd sentences appeared out of nowhere – babbling and a stupid grin prevailed. Trying desperately to gather myself and identify the mechanism by which I had lost all 'coolness', I reasoned that I was in this state due to the electricity, chemistry and uncertainty about what would happen next.

Over the next hour or two, the tension became too great. Not only was I not making sense, I had also begun to sweat. Granted it was a warm day, but certainly not to the extent where you look like you're running a marathon. At this point, I was desperate to keep it together and suggested a drink, as any form of sedation was now an urgent requirement. She enthusiastically agreed, however surprising it was that she was still on this date!

If I knew then what I know now, and that is that alcohol spikes

adrenalin and cortisol, I would have done things somewhat differently. Not only was my decision to have a drink far from the
appropriate action under the frenzied circumstances, but my
choice of beverage and speed of consumption further fuelled an
already chaotic situation.

Premium vodka, although free of congeners,[94] did not provide
the anticipated stabilising effect; rather, it amplified the excitement, uncertainty, joy, confusion and uncontainable chemistry. I
can only describe the experience as like playing tennis on a round-
about during a hurricane while trying to write a biology exam.

All these super-charged emotions combined with alcohol were
further fuelling my stress axis. It felt as if I was producing litres of
cortisol and adrenalin at that point. I could feel my heart pounding. I was still perspiring, but the adrenalin-mediated release of
endorphins was inducing a state of euphoria.

In a moment of banter, this woman of my dreams asked me
what her name was. For the life of me, I couldn't imagine why she
would ask something so obvious! After all, I had been fixating on
her for weeks already, to the extent that the world had ceased to
exist outside of her.

Here's the thing – under normal circumstances my memory and
recollection of facts, events and minute detail is fairly robust. Some
would even say that I have a photographic memory. However, with
super-physiological levels of cortisol, I honestly had no clue what
her name was! I played for time with the usual stalling strategies. I
repeated the question, asked her to rephrase the question and even
claimed that the scenario was nothing short of an interrogation, but I
was caught out. The date that I had been waiting for all my life ended
unceremoniously and with a great deal of animosity on her part.

She eventually forgave me following days of eloquent clarifi-
cation of the underlying hormonal mechanisms that induced my

transient amnesia. We were married a year later, and the event was included as part of my wedding speech.

The message here is that cortisol elevations, whether acute or over protracted periods, can be exceptionally detrimental within the cognitive domain, and any safe, non-toxic supplement that can reverse this phenomenon may prove invaluable.

Bacopa monnieri enhances cognition during stressful periods

In 2016, a team of researchers from the US and various centres in India published a study investigating the effectiveness of *Bacopa monnieri* in enhancing cognitive functionality over a six-week period (259). The study was a randomised, double-blind, placebo-controlled trial that involved 60 male and female medical students between the ages of 19 and 22. According to the authors, the decision to perform the study on medical students was strategic in that they are highly intelligent. Numerous research papers show that *Bacopa monnieri* is effective in general and ageing populations, but the question was whether *Bacopa monnieri* could influence this sub-set of the adult population.

Exclusion criteria were stringent to ensure a high level of accuracy. Participants had to refrain from taking medications and consuming alcohol as well as any other central nervous system stimulants. Moreover, the group had to be free of chronic diseases and not have used *Bacopa monnieri* before.

The outcome of the study clearly showed that supplementing with *Bacopa monnieri* at a dose of 300 mg per day dramatically enhanced attention, resulted in less distraction and improved working memory across multiple domains, both in the medium and short term.

Although *Bacopa monnieri's* powerful antioxidant effect and its influence on neurotransmitter[95] levels are believed to be the primary drivers in enhanced cognition as a result of supplementation, there appears to be far more to the story.

Bacosides A and B are unique constituents of *Bacopa monnieri*. Recent research shows that these compounds improve the transmission of impulses between nerve cells (259). Bacosides facilitate the regeneration of connections between nerve cells as well as repair damaged nerve cells. The combined effect of improved nerve communication, regeneration and repair is yet another reason why *Bacopa monnieri* has such a profound effect on memory and cognition.

Bacopa monnieri improves behaviour and cognition in children with ADHD and hyperactivity disorders

Not only does *Bacopa monnieri* promote memory formation and learning in adult populations, recent evidence shows that adolescent populations may also derive benefit through supplementation, specifically in terms of cognition and behaviour.

In 2016, *Complementary Therapies in Medicine* published a systematic review of the literature in child and adolescent populations (260).

The results demonstrated significant and consistent improvements in language, behaviour and cognitive functionality, as well as in the memory subdomains. However, what was particularly evident was the value that *Bacopa monnieri* had in improving hyperactivity and attention-deficit disorders.

One of the highlights of the review was that *Bacopa monnieri* is very well tolerated, with less than 2.5% of the participants experiencing only mild side effects, which were predominantly gastrointestinal.

Bacopa monnieri can protect the body from many of the adverse internal changes that result from stress

Some animal studies also suggest that *Bacopa monnieri* can profoundly influence the stress axis. A research article published in *Pharmacology, Biochemistry and Behavior* (261) showed *Bacopa monnieri* to be systemically protective under both chronic and acute stress conditions. The research team discovered that a major stressful event results in rapid biological adaptations that include increased adrenal gland weight, ulcerations in the stomach, higher blood glucose and a reduction in spleen weight. Consider that the spleen is a vital organ that has numerous functional roles that include immune regulation, blood filtration, and even storing a significant blood reserve.

> In nature, the default is always to survival. When confronted with major stressful events, our bodies instantly adapt. Changes take place in our organs – they can shrink or enlarge – hormonal levels rise or fall, and our immune system lies at the heart of these considerable adaptations. No area of our body is left unaffected by the ravages of stress.
>
> This is why it is imperative that we take regular preventative action to help our bodies regain their balance and physiological stability.

Chronic stress was shown to have an even more magnified effect on numerous biological systems. The researchers found that the adrenal glands were enlarged, blood glucose was elevated, stomach ulcerations were present, liver markers were raised and there was significant spleen shrinkage. There were also additional biological shifts that included alterations in blood lipids, raised cholesterol and a reduced thymus gland[96] weight. Reduced functionality of this specialised lymphoid organ results in immunosuppression and a high susceptibility to infection. As an adult, reduced thymus gland size is less impactful due in part to the fact that it begins to shrink during our teen years, and is not especially functional in adult life. However, should this gland become compromised as a child due to chronic stress or genetic abnormalities, the ramifications are enormous in the context of immune functionality both as an adolescent and later as an adult.

Remarkably, this study showed that pre-treatment with varying doses of *Bacopa monnieri* prior to acute stress simulations offset all of the negative biological adaptations, including the pathological reduction in spleen weight and enlargement of the adrenal glands. In the case of chronic stress, only a pre-treatment with a high dose was able to offset many of the negative biological adaptations, including stomach ulcer index, adrenal enlargement and liver markers.

According to the authors at the Central Drug Research Institute in India:

> *On the basis of our result, it is concluded that the standardised extract of* B. monnieri *possesses a potent adaptogenic activity.*

Bacopa monnieri reduces pain

Several recent studies are showing that *Bacopa monnieri* may also be effective in improving the symptoms of depression and pain. Researchers from the Department of Pharmacology at Bombay College of Pharmacy in India explored the possible mechanisms behind the strong pain-reducing effects of *Bacopa monnieri* using a variety of doses (262). The researchers discovered that the pain-reducing effects were not through one, but multiple interrelated pathways. According to the study, the pain-relieving effects are mediated by adrenalin, serotonin and natural opioids (endorphins).

This is not the only study focusing on pain reduction. In 2013, *Current Medicinal Chemistry* published a study on *Bacopa monnieri* as an emerging class of therapeutics in the management of chronic pain (263). The article highlights several important relationships, including that between depression and pain. According to this study, 77% of people experiencing chronic pain suffer from depression. Not only did the team of multinational researchers highlight the strong antidepressant and pain-modulating effects, they also compared its effects to morphine. In short, *Bacopa monnieri* is as effective in managing chronic pain as morphine. The paper highlights *Bacopa monnieri's* strong anti-inflammatory actions – which act along the same pathway as medications such as aspirin and ibuprofen – as making this naturally occurring plant particularly effective in managing nerve-related pain.

Current dosage guidelines

The standard dose is 300 mg per day, provided the active ingredients (bacosides) make up 55% of the dry weight. Note that:

- *Bacopa monnieri* is fat-soluble and requires a lipoid transporter to be absorbed. Therefore, it should be taken with a meal containing a high proportion of fats.[97]
- *Bacopa monnieri* is very well tolerated, with few known side effects. The only reported side effect is stomach upset, which can be reduced by consuming *Bacopa monnieri* with food.
- *Bacopa monnieri* acts synergistically with numerous adaptogens and nutrients, including ashwagandha, curcumin and catechins.[98]

Green tea and its role in stress resilience

I have been a huge fan of green tea for several years now. Hardly a day goes by when I don't have my two to three cups. It's probably no surprise that my interest in tea dates back to my time living in China, but over the years I have begun to fully appreciate the value that green tea holds in keeping me healthy, especially during periods of high demand.

While the more popular choice has traditionally been black tea, both green and black tea influence health and cognitive functionality through several molecular channels – albeit with varied effectiveness. Despite their differences, both teas are derived from the same plant – *Camellia sinensis*. The only difference between the two is how they are processed after harvesting. Green tea hardly undergoes any processing whatsoever, whereas black tea is fermented through exposure to microorganisms for a period of 6 to 12 months. Not only does the fermentation process affect flavour and appearance, it has also been shown to lower black tea's antioxidant and health-promoting potential. For this reason, this chapter focuses exclusively on green tea as a tool in chronic stress management and resilience.

The consumption of green tea in China and other parts of eastern Asia dates back thousands of years. Tea has been used traditionally for both medicinal purposes and the promotion of health. Because regular green tea is 99.9% water, it is non-caloric yet contains several powerful compounds, including polyphenols[99] and caffeine. The polyphenols found in green tea have been shown to offer protection to the biological systems that are most compromised during periods of chronic stress – the nervous and cardiovascular systems.

Green tea phytochemicals[100] are some of the strongest in the plant world. The two most influential of these phytochemicals are catechins (which include epicatechin, epigallocatechin, epicatechin gallate, and epigallocatechin gallate), and an amino acid that is almost exclusive to the tea plant, L-theanine.

Green tea catechins reduce the risk of stroke

A 2009 meta-analysis involving almost 200 000 participants pooled from nine studies (264) found that, regardless of their country of origin, persons who consumed three or more cups of tea per day had a 21% lower risk of suffering from a stroke than those consuming fewer than one cup per day. Although the results were clear, the team of researchers from the University of California's School of Medicine were not able to explain exactly why regular tea consumption promoted such profound health benefits.

While many experts who suggest that the benefits of green tea on the cardiovascular system and brain are due to its strong anti-inflammatory and antioxidant actions, there appears to be far more to green tea's cardiovascular influence, which science has recently uncovered. One thing has become increasingly clear – the catechins are a major contributor to the protective effects of green tea on the nervous and cardiovascular systems.

A study published in the *European Journal of Cardiovascular Prevention and Rehabilitation* (265) showed that catechins promote more than just protection of the cardiovascular system; they also improve functionality by facilitating improved blood delivery to the brain and heart. Despite this important discovery, even more has been discovered about the effect of catechins on the nervous and cardiovascular systems.

In 2016, a review published in *Molecules* (266) provided a detailed description of the numerous mechanisms that make catechins so effective in preventing cardiovascular compromise and disease. The research team from the Hubei University of Technology in China described how catechins are able to regulate fat metabolism by reducing existing levels of body fat, as well as reducing lipids found in the bloodstream and liver. Moreover, catechins were found to alter blood lipid metabolism thereby inhibiting the development of atherosclerosis and reducing the accumulation of cholesterol. Catechins also protect the blood vessel walls[101] from damage and can positively influence nitric oxide release[102] in the circulatory system. Lastly, catechins stabilise blood pressure and can even lower blood pressure in persons with hypertension.

The fact that regular consumption of green tea can reduce the risk of a stroke by 21% is profoundly significant, especially in terms of stress resilience. The reason is that the risk of having a stroke is dramatically elevated in response to chronic stress, particularly when coupled with long working hours – something few of us can avoid in this day and age.

In 2015, *The Lancet* published a study (5) on the relationship between the stress associated with long working hours and the impact that it has on health. The researchers analysed volumes of data from studies involving over 600 000[103] subjects and found that when compared with standard working hours,[104] those who worked in excess of 55 hours per week increased their risk of having a stroke by 33%. There was also a significantly increased risk of developing heart disease.

If three or more cups of green tea seems a lot, the good news is that in order to protect the cardiovascular and nervous systems, only two cups may be necessary. This finding comes off the back of a review of the literature by a Dutch team of researchers (267), which showed that 500 ml[105] of tea per day was associated with a dramatic increase in arterial diameter and significantly enhanced blood flow throughout the body. The reason for this is the effect of green tea catechins on increasing nitric oxide bioavailability and/or production (268).

L-theanine protects blood vessels

The L-theanine in green tea also offers considerable cardiovascular and neurological protection. An advantage of this unique protein is that it is highly bioavailable and is even able to permeate the brain's protective barrier, thereby positively influencing our brain waves and neurochemistry.

L-theanine makes up around 2% of the dry weight of tea, meaning that regular consumption can have a significant effect on circulating levels. L-theanine protects against arterial damage through a variety of channels, which include reduction in cholesterol production, improved dilatation of the arterial system, as well as increased nitric oxide production (269). This is another possible reason for the lower incidence of strokes found in persons who regularly consume green tea. The amazing thing is that studies on blood vessel compromise in the brain have reliably demonstrated that L-theanine has a neuroprotective effect, even at low dosages (270).

The dynamic duo in green tea (catechins and L-theanine) gives the brain a boost

Green tea consumption enhances not only the cardiovascular system, but also the brain. More and more research is showing that green tea polyphenols potentiate the action of BDNF, thereby promoting improved structural integrity and functionality of the brain. According to researchers in the Department of Cell and Neurobiology and the Department of Pharmacology and Pharmaceutical Sciences at the University of Southern California (271), the main protagonist in improved BDNF potentiation is the catechin epigallocatechin-3-gallate (EGCG). According to the study, this phenomenal effect requires only the smallest amount of EGCG.

Another way in which our cognitive and behavioural state may be enhanced through regular consumption of green tea is through the positive influence of L-theanine on the neurochemicals dopamine and serotonin. A Japanese study published in *Neurochemical Research* (272) showed that L-theanine increases serotonin and dopamine and optimises their metabolism within key regions of the brain.[106] These findings have been replicated in more recent studies.

The collective effect of serotonin and dopamine includes improvements in attention, focus, concentration, learning, memory, mood, muscle contraction, bone metabolism, coordination, cardiovascular function, digestion and sleep.

The improvements in cognitive functionality associated with green tea consumption are not effected exclusively through improved potentiation of BDNF and the influence on dopamine and serotonin, but also through alterations in actual brain wave behaviour.

L-theanine has been shown to increase the propensity to being in an alpha brain wave state, in much the same way as various forms of meditation and aerobic exercise do. This frequency is represented by a state of relaxation, and essentially bridges the gap between our conscious thinking mind and our subconscious.

Alpha waves promote greater mental coordination, calmness, a state of restful alertness, better mind/body integration, as well as potential for improved learning.

When we become chronically stressed, alpha brain waves become less prevalent, leading to a reduced ability to cope, anxiety, obsessive behaviours and insomnia.

Research published in the *Korean Journal of Nutrition* (273) as well as *Trends in Food Science and Technology* (274) showed that L-theanine crosses the blood-brain barrier within 30 minutes of intake and increases activity in the alpha frequency band of the electroencephalogram (EEG). Like the biological changes seen with L-theanine, relatively small amounts are able to positively alter brain waves in a way that promotes not only relaxation, but also creates greater neurological flexibility.

L-theanine and the stress response

In 2007, *Biological Psychology* (275) published a study that investigated the effects of L-theanine on the body during periods of stress. This small Japanese trial clearly showed that L-theanine intake during periods of stress resulted in a reduction in heart rate and a more stable immune response to an acute stress task relative to the placebo control group. The authors surmised that L-theanine could promote significant anti-stress effects by lowering excitation[107] of the nervous system. Simply put, L-theanine can put the brakes on the first wave of the stress response, creating better biological behaviours in response to life's challenges.

Animal studies also suggest that L-theanine intake can lower stress hormone concentrations[108] both at rest and in response to stress (276), creating a less damaging and more balanced biological state. Simply put, L-theanine moderates the second wave of the stress response.

With both waves of the stress response moderated, L-theanine has one more special feature with respect to stress – it can repair the damage caused by chronic exposure. Researchers from the Xuzhou Medical College in Jiangsu, China, found (277) that L-theanine treatment can reverse the cognitive impairment and neurological damage that result from protracted stress. Substantiating the previously cited studies, L-theanine lowered abnormal levels of stress hormones and positively influenced the neurochemicals dopamine and serotonin.

Is timing of L-theanine intake important for stress resilience?

With many stress-buffering practices, there is an art to timing the intervention to achieve the maximum desired effect. The question is whether the same model applies to the consumption of L-theanine-rich green tea. Researchers at the Nagoya University Department of Psychology in Japan (275) evaluated a small group of participants under simulated psychological stress, either with or without L-theanine supplementation. The participants were divided into four groups:

- Group 1 took L-theanine at the start of the experiment
- Group 2 took L-theanine midway
- Group 3 was a control group that took an identical placebo
- Group 4 was a control group that took nothing.

The results showed that L-theanine intake, irrespective of timing, resulted in a reduction in the negative biological effects of the stress response, specifically in the context of neurological, hormonal and immune markers. In short, whether you have your green tea before the day starts or in the middle of the chaos, the benefit is the same!

Caffeine is a powerful nootrophic

It is common knowledge that caffeine[109] is a powerful stimulant, and that it can be used to improve physical strength and endurance. It is also classified as a nootropic[110] because it sensitises brain cells and provides tremendous mental stimulation.

It is fair to say that many people in industrialised nations are addicted to its mentally stimulating effects. Whether we drink it to get up in the morning, get through the day, or to increase our mental alertness, its role in society is nothing short of a full-blown dependency, myself included!

Fortunately, unless you consume more than 400 mg per day, which amounts to more than 3 cups of coffee (or more than 10 to 12 cups of green tea), or you have a medical condition[111] for which caffeine is contra-indicated, it is safe and, in some instances, even health promoting.

That said, I would like to emphasise moderation! The reason is that caffeine in excess can trigger the stress axis, sending your body into overdrive.

Research has shown that caffeine enhances cognitive performance in a variety of settings. A randomised, double-blind, placebo-controlled trial performed on 60 participants at the University of Missouri in St Louis (277a) showed that when compared to a placebo, caffeine intake significantly improved sustained attention, cognitive effort and reaction times in healthy adults.

Evidence also indicates a general improvement in the ability to accommodate new and relevant information within working memory, as well as overall enhanced brain activation.

Excess caffeine sends the stress axis into overdrive

A 2008 study to investigate the hormonal effects of caffeine, published in the *International Journal of Sport Nutrition and Exercise Metabolism* (278), found that high doses of caffeine[112] increased cortisol levels by 52%. This was not an isolated finding. At least three other randomised control trials have reported similar results.

Cortisol is not the only stress hormone that is elevated in response to excess caffeine consumption. Adrenalin is also affected. A randomised, double-blind, crossover study involving a small group of healthy volunteers (279) showed that high caffeine consumption resulted in a five-fold increase in adrenalin concentrations in the bloodstream. At least two other studies have reported similar findings, indicating a high degree of corroboration in the literature.

Lastly, in 2013, *Behavioural Brain Research* (280) published a study showing that psychosocial stress, combined with the equivalent of two to four cups of strong coffee,[113] was associated with a 233% enhanced adrenalin release and a 211% enhanced cortisol release when compared to placebo conditions.

> The essence of resilience is balance through biological modulation. Excessive caffeine intake does the exact opposite! It spikes cortisol by 52% and it increases adrenalin production fivefold. When you're highly stressed, excess caffeine will significantly amplify your immediate experience.

Green tea is completely safe

Fortunately, there is little or no risk of exposing yourself to excessive caffeine with green tea. A typical cup of green tea contains ±25–29 mg of caffeine whereas a strong filter coffee can have as much as 160 mg. Although an espresso seems strong due to its concentrated form, the caffeine content is far lower than a filter coffee (50–60 mg). You would have to drink well over 3 litres of green tea to expose yourself to excess caffeine, but more importantly,

L-theanine in green tea balances the effects of caffeine, thereby neutralising any potential risk.

L-theanine and caffeine, a cognitive powerhouse

When caffeine is combined with L-theanine, they significantly improve several aspects of memory and attention. A 2008 study published in *Nutritional Neuroscience* (271) compared the effects of caffeine, caffeine with L-theanine, and a placebo on several aspects of working memory and attention. Here is what they found:

- When taken on its own, caffeine's effect was compartmentalised. For example, 60 minutes after caffeine consumption, response speed to mentally demanding challenges improved. Thirty minutes later, accuracy with the cognitive challenges improved. In other words, only one aspect improves at a time.
- When L-theanine and caffeine were combined, both response speed and accuracy improved 60 minutes after ingestion and were sustained throughout the series of mental challenges.

Since the ability to focus attention requires speed and accuracy, this suggests that the combination found in green tea could be far superior to caffeine on its own, as found in coffee and energy drinks.

The stress-buffering effects of cacao/cocoa

Both cacao and cocoa are derived from the seeds of the cacao tree – *Theobroma cacao*. The difference between the two is simply that cocoa has undergone heating and processing, which may affect the flavonoid content slightly. Originally found only in the Americas, indigenous cultures have consumed cacao and cocoa products for their curative and health-promoting properties for thousands of years.

Recently, the demand for cocoa beans has skyrocketed, not for their broad range of medicinal properties, but because our society is obsessed with chocolate – and rightly so. I say this because not only is chocolate delicious, it can also be good for you. You will soon find out why.

Because cacao is in a more natural state, it should be your first choice, where possible. Cacao contains more than 300 constituents. In fact, its array of health-promoting phytochemicals is nothing short of astonishing. Many of the acclaimed health benefits are derived from the broad range of polyphenols, including catechins, procyanidins, clovamide, cinnamtannin, quercetin, and resveratrol. In their own right, each of these compounds has the potential to counteract the negative effects of protracted stress. As a collective, the benefits supersede mere stabilisation of health – they may even offer performance enhancement.

Cacao contains the stimulants caffeine and theobromine, as well as compounds that positively influence several neurochemicals, including dopamine and norepinephrine.

As if the array of health-promoting polyphenols wasn't enough, consider that cacao shoots the lights out in the antioxidant department. According to a 2011 research study published in the *Chemistry Central Journal* (281), cacao has one of the highest antioxidant profiles in the plant kingdom, completely outperforming blueberries, acai berries, and other renowned superfoods.

The epicatechin in cacao offers protection against several modern diseases
As is the case with green tea, the epicatechins found in cacao are capturing the attention of researchers, and for good reason. A few years ago, *ScienceDaily* (282) reported that epicatechins rival prominent antibiotics and anaesthesia in terms of their importance to public health.

This statement comes off the back of extensive research by Dr Norman Hollenberg, a professor of Medicine at Harvard Medical School. Hollenberg has spent years studying the remarkable health profiles of the Kuna people in Panama. He found that the risk of four of the most common killer diseases[114] – stroke, heart failure, cancer and diabetes – is reduced to less than 10%

in this unique group. After taking several factors into account, including environment, genetics, stress, pollution and diet, Hollenberg surmised that their secret weapon in disease prevention was their high intake of cacao. His study found that the Kuna people can drink up to 40 cups of cocoa a week, thus ingesting copious amounts of epicatechin, not to mention other health-promoting flavonoids. In fact, according to Hollenberg's research paper entitled "Flavanols, the Kuna, cocoa consumption and nitric oxide" (283), the Kuna are probably the highest flavonol-consuming community on Earth.

According to the study, the mechanism by which cocoa consumption positively influences health is by activating nitric oxide synthesis.[115]

These findings have been so well received by the scientific community that randomised controlled trials may well be the next step.

According to Hollenberg:

> If these observations predict the future, then we can say without blushing that they are among the most important observations in the history of medicine. We all agree that penicillin and anaesthesia are enormously important. But epicatechin could potentially get rid of four of the five most common diseases in the western world, how important does that make epicatechin? ... I would say very important.

Leading authorities on health will continue to probe epicatechin to find ways to bring its health-promoting properties to bear on various global health challenges. What we can take from this is the value of epicatechin within a broader stress resilience model. The reason is that cardiovascular and neurological issues are at the forefront of chronic stress – foods that can offer protection against these consequences should be considered invaluable.

The quercetin in cacao/cocoa lowers biological stress

Not only does the epicatechin in cacao/cocoa positively influence our health and protect us from the effects of chronic stress, cacao/cocoa contains another flavonoid that warrants a standing ovation – the plant pigment quercetin. Quercetin is the 'super' in many of the known superfoods[116] – they are loaded with this unique plant pigment.

In 2010, Japanese researchers (284) published an animal study showing that quercetin[117] supplementation was able to stabilise and balance[118] the body's response to extreme stress. The study found that with aggressive stress simulations, the lab rats given high doses of quercetin experienced stress hormone suppression[119] as well as positive genetic changes that promoted greater biological stability under harsh and testing conditions.

In the same year, another animal study published in the *European Journal of Pharmacology* (285) reported almost identical findings.[120] What was interesting about this study is that it pointed out that quercetin enters the brain within several hours of ingestion and has a positive and direct effect on brain cells. The researchers discovered that quercetin reverses the free radical damage caused by stress in the hypothalamus, a region of the brain that controls and regulates the stress axis.

The study points out that chronic stress is associated with the production of several damaging compounds in the brain, including several types of harmful free radicals, one of which is lipid hydroperoxide. Additionally, stress is associated with the depletion of key antioxidant enzymes. The combined effect of higher free radicals and lower antioxidant enzymes results in significant structural damage. Remarkably, quercetin has been shown to scavenge free radicals as well as inhibit lipid hydroperoxides, thereby offering a high degree of neuroprotection. The authors concluded by stating that quercetin may be an effective tool in the prevention and treatment of stress-induced oxidative damage in the brain.

Good news for dark chocolate lovers
Recently, Swiss researchers (286) set out to investigate whether a single administration of dark chocolate buffers hormonal responses to stress. Moreover, the team from the University of Bern wanted to determine whether this

effect would be at the level of the adrenal glands[121] or principally within the brain.[122]

The trial was placebo-controlled and involved healthy, medication-free, non-smoking men between the ages of 20 and 50. The dark chocolate used in the study contained 281 kcal and 125 mg of epicatechin per 50 g serving. The placebo chocolate contained 310 kcal and no epicatechin per 50 g serving. The placebo was a flavonoid-free, white chocolate that was dyed and flavoured to match the colour, appearance and smell of the dark chocolate.

All the participants were subjected to stress simulations. This involved a five-minute mock job interview and a five-minute mental arithmetic task in front of an audience two hours after chocolate ingestion, when the plasma flavonoid levels were expected to peak.

The blood and saliva samples that were taken at various points during the study revealed that prior to the simulation, there were no differences between the treatment group (ingesting epicatechin-rich, dark chocolate) and the placebo group. Across all participants, the stress test induced significant increases in cortisol, ACTH, epinephrine and norepinephrine. However, the dark-chocolate group showed a significantly blunted cortisol (30% less) and adrenalin (15% less) reactivity to psychosocial stress when compared with the placebo group. There were no group differences in terms of ACTH or norepinephrine stress reactivity. The researchers also found that the higher the epicatechin levels, the lower the cortisol and adrenalin spikes in response to stress.

This study clearly shows that cacao/cocoa flavanols affect the stress axis at the level of the adrenal glands. The impact of this essentially means a dramatically reduced burden on a system (adrenals) that is completely over-taxed in this day and age.

Two years later, the same team of researchers published a study highlighting the effects of flavanol-rich, dark chocolate on systemic inflammation, a major issue attributed to chronic stress. The 2016 study (287) highlighted that the epicatechins found in cacao/cocoa blunted the elevated immune response to stress, both in terms of the primary driver[123] and the molecules that promote inflammation.[124] Like the previous study, the results showed that higher intakes of cacao/cocoa flavanols were associated with greater responses.

Around 50 g of dark chocolate – preferably containing over 75% cocoa – can significantly reduce cortisol, adrenalin and inflammation when consumed prior to stressful events or challenges. How can we say no to that?

Cacao/cocoa[125] boosts brain power

There has also been significant interest in cacao/cocoa's effect on cognition, memory and behaviour. Part of the reason for the scientific community's attention in this space is certainly epicatechin, but also other more psycho-active components of cacao/cocoa, which include methylxanthines, caffeine and theobromine. All of these constituents have been correlated with improvements in alertness and cognitive function (288).

It's hard to believe that just a single intake of cacao/cocoa, whether in a healthy treat, a piece or two of dark chocolate, or even in the protein shake recipe given at the end of this section, can have an almost immediate effect. Yet it does! In fact, there is considerable evidence of noticeable improvements in cognitive function following a single dose of dark chocolate (or cacao/cocoa flavanols). According to a randomised, placebo-controlled, double-blind, balanced, three-period crossover trial on 30 healthy adults published in the *Journal of Psychopharmacology* (289), improvements in information processing speed and working memory can be observed within hours of cacao/cocoa flavanol consumption. Several other studies report similar findings.

Cacao/cocoa protects the brain from ageing

Not only does cacao/cocoa positively influence short-term cognition, it also has the potential to slow the rate of cognitive decline that occurs as a result of ageing. This is relevant because chronic stress accelerates the ageing process in the body, and especially in the brain. Could a few squares of dark chocolate protect us against age-related decline? According to the research evidence, it appears that it can.

In 2015, Italian researchers conducted a dietary intervention study (290) on the long-term effects of cocoa flavanols. Prior to the eight-week, double-blind, placebo-controlled dietary intervention, the 90 elderly participants performed several mental acuity tests, which were repeated at the end of the study. Incredibly, eight weeks of daily cocoa consumption resulted in significantly improved test scores. Moreover, treatment groups consuming higher quantities of cocoa flavanols showed greater overall improvements.

A cross-sectional analysis of 968 participants in the US (291) revealed that habitual polyphenol-rich chocolate intake was related to improved cognitive performance, as measured by an extensive battery of neuropsychological tests. More frequent chocolate consumption was associated with significantly better performance in terms of:

- visual-spatial memory
- organisation
- working memory
- scanning and tracking, and
- abstract reasoning.

All these aspects of cognition are impacted by chronic stress. Before you pile into slabs of dark chocolate in the hope of preserving your brain or protecting it from the ravages of chronic stress, just be mindful that more research needs to be done to substantiate these findings and provide optimal consumption guidelines that take sugar content and processing into account. Nevertheless, it is certainly an exciting space for those who have been subjected to protracted periods of chronic stress and are feeling cognitively compromised.

How does cacao/cocoa affect our brains?

There have been several proposed mechanisms by which these powerful flavanols from the cacao/cocoa bean directly impact cognition and, potentially, behaviour. It is thought that the driving forces are the antioxidant, anti-inflammatory and insulin-lowering effects, but there appear to be others.

A German review entitled "Chocolate and the brain: neurobiological impact of cocoa flavanols on cognition and behaviour" (292) investigated how cocoa flavanols promote brain performance and why they offer significant neuroprotection, especially during periods of stress. The researchers identified several important pathways:

1. When consuming cacao or cocoa-rich foods, the flavonoids are absorbed rapidly. Within 30 minutes they can be detected in the bloodstream and will peak between two and three hours after intake. Incidentally, levels return to baseline six to eight hours after ingestion.

2. Once absorbed, the flavanols cross the blood-brain barrier and accumulate in the regions of the brain involved in learning and memory. Flavanols are known to have direct interactions with the cellular component that increases the expression of BDNF.[126]

3. Cacao/cocoa flavanols increase cerebral blood flow as well as blood perfusion throughout the entire central and peripheral nervous systems. The higher blood flow increases the supply of oxygen and glucose to the billions of neurons in the brain, and is associated with better removal of waste products, not only in the brain, but also in other sensory systems. Incredibly not only is blood flow enhanced where we need it most during stress, but the actual blood supply network is reinforced. According to a 2007 animal study published in the *Journal of Neuroscience* (293), epicatechin administration stimulates the formation of new blood vessels[127] in the hippocampus.

While these insights clearly identify the long-term actions of cacao/cocoa flavanols in counteracting oxidative stress, neuro-inflammation and neuro-degeneration, the exact mechanisms of the more immediate improvements in brain function and behaviour have yet to be fully understood.

Cacao/cocoa protects and enhances the cardiovascular system

Earlier chapters describe the impact of stress-induced adrenalin spikes on the blood vessels of the brain and heart. Several large studies involving hundreds of thousands of participants have shown that the risk of having a stroke or heart attack increases substantially during chronic stress (by 33% and 27% respectively).

Cacao/cocoa flavanols have been shown to mitigate the cardiovascular risks through a variety of different channels. Again, making positive changes to our bodies via many channels means that the intervention really works.

One of the first large studies investigating cocoa intake and the effects on the cardiovascular system was published in the *Archives of Internal Medicine* in 2006 (294). The study included 470 Dutch men who were free of cardiovascular disease and diabetes. The study found that after an adjustment for a wide range of possible external influences that could affect the results, both systolic and diastolic blood pressure were inversely associated with cocoa intake. Simply put, participants who consumed more cocoa had healthier blood pressure profiles and greater protection from cardiovascular diseases. The study also revealed that cocoa consumption was associated with a lower risk of premature mortality, especially from cardiovascular compromise. When comparisons were made between those who consumed the most cocoa in their diet and those who consumed the least, the rates of cardiovascular disease and premature mortality were 50% lower. If you currently don't have a history of cardiovascular problems, you can expect robust protection from cocoa-rich foods.

However, if chronic stress has already taken a toll on your cardiovascular system, cacao/cocoa flavanols may offer some much-needed protection. The current narrative supports the notion that cacao/cocoa flavanols offer cardiovascular protection to apparently healthy persons, but where the research really stands out is that it profoundly protects persons who already have a history of a significant cardiac event.

In 2009, a Swedish study on 1 169 participants assessed cardiac mortality in patients[128] hospitalised for their first heart attack. Patients self-reported dark chocolate consumption for the preceding 12 months and were monitored for hospitalisations and mortalities in the national registry for eight years. The study showed that the patients who reported eating dark chocolate two or more times per week were 66% less likely to suffer a cardiac death compared with those who reported never eating chocolate.

A final note on stress and cardiovascular disease

While it has been well established that stress is one of the most important lifestyle factors that can influence the incidence of cardiovascular disease, diet can be equally important. According to David Katz of the Yale University School of Medicine (295), cacao/cocoa and other flavonoids can lower stress-induced cardiovascular risk by protecting fats (lipids), proteins and even genetic material from oxidative damage, as well as by reducing inflammation and regulating blood vessel balance.

Cacao/cocoa intake

Although cacao is preferable to cocoa because it is less processed and there-fore contains a richer antioxidant/flavonoid profile, both offer significant health benefits.

Choosing your cacao/cocoa

- It is best to choose organic sources where possible.
- Excess sugar and food additives, such as flavourants and preservatives, can negate some of the benefits, so go for options that have as few of these ingredients as possible.

- Consuming dairy products with cocoa-rich foods – specifically milk and cheese – may interfere with flavonoid absorption (296). The reason appears to be related to a protein found in dairy products known as casein. It is highly unlikely that a whey protein concentrate or isolate would have this effect.
- You can add cacao/cocoa to smoothies, porridge, and homemade snacks as a healthy alternative to commercially produced confectionaries and sweets.
- Dark chocolate is a really good source of cocoa flavanols. Typically, 5–26 g of dark chocolate contains anywhere from 65 mg to 1095 mg of flavanols. Part of the reason for the variance is the percentage of cocoa in the product – today we can get chocolate with 70%, 85%, or even over 99% cocoa! The other factor is the quality of the cocoa itself.
- To get the ideal amount of cocoa flavanols from dark chocolate, consuming 25–40 g of 85% cocoa or above (if you have the palate), would be perfect.
- Taken as a supplement,[129] the ideal dose would be 500–1000 mg per day taken with meals.
- To date no ideal prescriptive dose in terms of amount or frequency has been fully established for cacao and cocoa-containing foods. Until such time as guidelines are put forward, it may be wise to stay on the moderate side of cacao/cocoa consumption.

Try the delicious, healthy breakfast or snack recipe on the next page to boost your brain power.

Brain boosting chocolate smoothie

2.5 tablespoons raw cacao or cocoa (organic if possible)

1 tablespoon cacao nibs

6–8 heaped tablespoons of pure whey protein isolate powder

(free of lactose (<1%) and casein)

1 tablespoon of almond or cashew nut butter[130]

1 tablespoon pumpkin seeds

1 tablespoon chia seeds

1 tablespoon flax seeds

10 walnut halves

4 large dates (remove pits)

150–400 ml cold water or almond milk (amount depends on

personal preference regarding consistency)

Two cups of ice

Add all ingredients together in a blender and blend till smooth.

Serves two to three.

CHAPTER SUMMARY

- Rebuilding and repairing the damage caused by chronic stress is indeed possible. And it's true to say that the work you do to become healthy and stress resilient will serve you well in the future. Your lifestyle changes will protect you from the severe biological and psychological effects of chronic stress, no matter what challenges life brings.
- Restoration of the vitality, health and cognitive potency lost through chronic stress can be achieved through numerous sustained lifestyle behaviours and practices.

- The key to neutralising the long-term effects of stress is to focus on the very hormones and molecules that become down-regulated by the two waves in the stress response, most importantly brain-derived neurotrophic factor and other neurotrophins, growth hormone, and the neurotransmitters serotonin and dopamine.
- Many activities, nutritional supplements (nutraceuticals), dietary practices, and being outdoors can increase the production and circulating levels of several of these molecules and hormones.
- The lifestyle practices in this chapter will enhance cognitive potential, emotional stability and physical integrity. These include:
- **Exercise routines** that improve functionality and structure of the brain, and that promote hormonal shifts that strengthen and enhance our physical vitality.
- **Dietary interventions such as caloric restriction and intermittent fasting** that will improve hormonal integrity and lower inflammation, as well as enhance genetic behaviour favouring health, youth and vitality.
- **Sunlight exposure** that is safe and promotes cognitive and behavioural improvements, and provides cardiovascular protection, immune enhancement and improved genetic functionality.
- **Supplements** ranging from caloric restriction mimetics, such as curcumin and resveratrol, to multivitamins, B-complex and omega-3 fatty acids, all of which positively influence the stress axis, promote speedier recovery from chronic stress and are instrumental in restoring health after prolonged allostatic load.
- **Curcumin:**
  - is a potent mimetic that provides the same physiological benefits as fasting and caloric restriction (see chapter for details)
  - has been used in Eastern medicine for more than 2 000 years to manage stress and brain-related ailments
  - has antioxidant, anti-inflammatory and anti-carcinogenic[131] effects

- offers protection from cardiovascular and neurological diseases
- stabilises BDNF levels in the brain during periods of chronic stress
- can be used successfully in the management of depression, and
- stabilises key neurotransmitters, such as serotonin, dopamine and norepinephrine during periods of stress.

■ **Resveratrol:**
- provides the same physiological benefits as fasting and caloric restriction
- positively alters the psychological and physical responses to stress
- can counter the negative biological effects of an overactive stress response
- increases the expression of BDNF, thereby improving brain structure and function
- increases the secretion of serotonin and norepinephrine, enhancing mood and cognition
- has the potential to protect the brain from chronic stress hormone exposure
- may be effective in the management of several neurodegenerative disorders.

■ **Multivitamins:**
- Research has shown that high-quality multivitamins significantly reduce the physical and psychological symptoms related to chronic stress.
- Research shows that a high quality multivitamin taken for a period of 1–3 months can:
  - Decrease perceived stress by 35%
  - Reduce anxiety by 32%
  - Lower stress-induced psychiatric symptoms by 30%, and
  - Improve self-reported levels of clarity and cognition by 23%.

■ Consider that no standard or regulatory definition for multivitamins currently exists. This means that product compositions are highly variable in terms of nutrients, quantities and quality.

■ **Safety:**
- According to the National Institutes of Health, taking a basic multi-vitamin supplement that provides nutrients close to conservative recommended intakes should pose no safety risks to healthy people.
- Higher doses of many vitamins and minerals over prolonged periods of time might not only be ineffectual, but also detrimental to your health. Less is always more!

■ **B vitamins:**
- The B vitamins are vital to the body's ability to produce energy, making them invaluable in promoting stress resilience
- Vitamins B6, B9 and B12 play a vital role in maintaining our health during periods of chronic stress by converting homocysteine (a highly toxic compound that is elevated in response to chronic stress), into beneficial methionine, thus preventing extensive damage to the cardiovascular and nervous systems.
- Chronic stress creates a greater demand for B vitamins while at the same time depleting them, resulting in deficiencies.
- Many of the adverse health effects of chronic stress can be attributed to deficiencies in vitamins B6, B9 and B12.
- B vitamins are important in the production of many neurochemicals that influence stress responses in the body. The slightest deficiencies can result in greater susceptibility and reactivity to stress as well as significant psychological and metabolic disorders.
- In the interests of long-term health and vitality, it is recommended that you always choose a high quality multivitamin or B-complex formulation over individual micro-nutrients.

■ **Omega-3 fatty acids:**
- are believed to be the single most important nutrient complex in the human diet

- □ can blunt cortisol and adrenalin output during periods of chronic stress
- □ protect brain cells from the damaging effects of cortisol
- □ supplementation offers greater biological benefits to those who suffer from higher degrees of stress
- □ supplementation improves cognition and increases brain mass
- □ lowers systemic inflammation, and
- □ ongoing consumption is linked to greater longevity and lower rates of chronic diseases.
- ■ **Adaptogens** (including *Rhodiola rosea*, ashwagandha and *Bacopa monnieri*) are a group of plant-derived compounds that are known to increase attention and endurance when we are in a state of fatigue. They:
  - □ are able to significantly reduce stress-induced impairments and disorders related to multiple systems, including the nervous, hormonal, cardiovascular and immune systems
  - □ enable the body to successfully adapt to numerous environmental conditions, and are able to prevent damage through better regulation of metabolism
  - □ are able to strongly influence the body's response to numerous neurochemicals and hormones, especially stress hormones, steroid hormones and even serotonin
  - □ can have multiple, sometimes overlapping, pharmacological and biological effects
  - □ act as a stress vaccine thereby promoting 'immunity' to more severe or protracted stress, and
  - □ reduce free radical production, increase energy production, and facilitate enhanced repair of damaged proteins.
- ■ **Green tea** contains two vitally important stress-buffering compounds: catechins and L-theanine.
- ■ These compounds improve functionality and protect both the

nervous and cardiovascular systems.

- They augment BDNF, increase dopamine and serotonin as well as positively influence brain waves.
- They possess strong stress-moderating effects by reducing physiological reactivity to life's challenges (i.e. your heart rate won't race as much, your cortisol will be less elevated and your immune reactions will be less acute).
- The combination of caffeine and L-theanine in green tea enhances cognition without evoking the stress axis and appreciably raising stress hormones.
- Consuming more than 2–4 cups of coffee a day (>400 mg of caffeine) has been shown to significantly elevate cortisol and adrenalin independently of a stress stimulus.
- Research shows that high levels of stress combined with excess coffee can raise cortisol levels by 233% and adrenalin by 211%. Raised stress hormones as a consequence of excess caffeine amplify our experience of stress and reduce our ability to cope.
- **Cacao/cocoa** is extremely rich in anti-oxidants and contains hundreds of health-promoting polyphenols.
  - Cacao/cocoa is particularly rich in epicatechin, a phytochemical that protects us from several stress-induced diseases.
  - Like green tea, cacao/cocoa also has the ability to stabilise the stress response by reducing cortisol and adrenalin output during life's challenges.
  - Cacao/cocoa promotes enhanced function and stability within the immune system.
  - There are numerous compounds found in cacao/cocoa that improve our cognitive abilities by increasing the levels of important neurochemicals in the brain.
  - Cacao/cocoa enhances the brain's structure and protects it from stress-induced damage as well as the ageing process.

- ◻ The cardiovascular system is enhanced and protected by the wide range of compounds found in cacao/cocoa.
- ▪ Collectively, green tea and cacao/cocoa enhance, strengthen and protect the three systems that are most impacted by chronic stress – immune, nervous and cardiovascular.

ALCOHOL

In itself, alcohol is a contentious issue in any health or social context, let alone in relation to chronic stress. While all researchers agree that over-consumption of alcohol is absolutely detrimental to health, there are very polarised camps with regard to moderate alcohol consumption in persons with no history of alcohol abuse. Several health organisations and research-ers believe that even light-to-moderate alcohol consumption offers no benefits whatsoever, and have shown that its relationship to health is nega-tive. Conversely, countless research papers show numerous positive health associations in moderate alcohol consumption. What makes this debate more confusing is that both sides of the divide are very well researched and substantiated.

This makes it very challenging for a health-conscious layperson to know who to believe and where to turn to for advice.

However, the moderate alcohol consumption debate becomes very real in the context of chronic stress – as changes in consumption and related behaviours show appreciable swings in this domain.

Although a glass of wine or a premium whiskey is not only enjoyable, but can offer perceived emotional and psychological respite from the chaos of life, it is important to realise that beyond moderate and occasional consumption, alcohol ingestion can actually amplify stress and impair coping mechanisms with devastating consequences.

As the following sections will show, my aim is not to elucidate the health debate, but rather to expose the negative relationship between alcohol and the stress axis.

■

THE ARGUMENT *AGAINST* MODERATE ALCOHOL CONSUMPTION

It has long been known that alcohol is a strong psychoactive substance with dependence-producing properties. Moreover, alcohol is a major global health issue, not to mention the burden it places on the world economy in terms of lost productivity and disability.

According to a 2014 WHO Global Status Report on Alcohol and Health (297), alcohol consumption in 2012 was directly attributed to 3.3 million deaths.

The same report highlighted that alcohol consumption contributes to more than 200 diseases and injury-related health conditions. These include liver cirrhosis, nutritional deficiencies, metabolic disturbances, several cancers, as well as physical injuries. Moreover, heavy use of alcohol ranks among the top five risk factors for disease, disability and death throughout the world.

Alcohol consumption carries with it the risk of abuse
One of the most significant issues with alcohol consumption is the potential for abuse and/or dependence. According to a 2015 National Survey on Drug Use and Health (298) in the US, over 6% of adults have an alcohol use disorder, many of whom have to undergo extensive rehabilitation. More concerning is the fact that 2.5% of children aged 12 to 17 are grappling with the same issue.

Strong genetic component in alcohol abuse behaviours

There is considerable evidence from human genetic studies that there is a strong hereditary component. According to a 2008 study entitled "Genetic approaches to addiction: genes and alcohol" (299), more than half of alcohol abuse disorders are genetically inherited. This is not to say that environmental factors don't play an equally important role in the development of alcohol-related disorders.

Alcohol consumption is linked to increased risk of certain cancers

In recent years, strong associations have been made between heavy alcohol consumption and certain cancers. According to a study published in the *British Medical Journal* (300), excessive alcohol consumption has been linked to intestinal, breast, mouth, throat, liver and oesophageal cancers. There is also evidence that heavy alcohol consumption may be linked to stomach, lung, gallbladder and pancreatic cancers.

While there is no medical debate about the relationship between heavy alcohol consumption and the elevated risk of cancer, the association between light-to-moderate alcohol consumption and cancer risk is less clear.

In 2015, Harvard researchers from the departments of Epidemiology and Nutrition published results from two large US studies (300). The objective of the paper was to quantify the risk of developing all types of cancers across all levels of alcohol consumption among women and men separately, with a focus on light-to-moderate drinking rather than heavy consumption. The participants' smoking histories were also included in the criteria.

A total of 135 965 men and women participated in the two studies, which were initiated in the 1980s and came to completion around 2010.

The studies showed that alcohol consumption above 30 g per day[1] was associated with an increased risk of developing many forms of cancer, particularly amongst participants with a history of smoking.

In men who had never smoked, the risk of alcohol-related cancers did not increase if they limited their number of drinks to two per day.

The same cannot be said for women – moderate alcohol consumption, even when combined with a history of never having smoked, correlated with an increased cancer risk, specifically breast cancer. The elevated risk in women was still present with intakes involving no more than one alcoholic drink a day. Whenever I give a talk on this topic to corporates, or executive teams, there is an audible sigh in the room and banter about the lack of fairness.

Your parents were right, long-term alcohol consumption may shrink your brain

Another area of debate is the effect of moderate alcohol consumption throughout life on the integrity of the brain and nervous system. In June of 2017, medical researchers at Oxford University published an observational group study (301), which had measured weekly alcohol intake and cognitive performance over a 30-year period. The study involved 550 participants with an average age of 43 when the study commenced. Not only did the study measure cognitive integrity and performance, it also used MRI scans to measure changes in brain structure.[2]

The results of this study showed that higher alcohol consumption over the 30-year period was associated with increased odds of brain shrinkage, especially in our memory centres, in a dose-dependent fashion. This means that the more alcohol we drink over a protracted period, the smaller our brains get. The question is: where is the tipping point in consumption or what is the threshold?

For the study, the measure of consumption was an alcohol unit, which equated to 10 ml or 8 g of pure alcohol. The researchers found that, compared with abstainers, participants who consumed more than 30 units[3] a week were the most susceptible to negative changes in brain structure and function. Even those who consumed alcohol to a degree of moderation[4] had a three-times higher risk of brain atrophy than abstainers. Generally speaking, 1–7 units per weeks did not have a major impact on neurological integrity.

THE ARGUMENT *FOR* MODERATE ALCOHOL CONSUMPTION

Despite the abundance of evidence suggesting that abstaining from alcohol promotes better health and overall well-being, there are numerous high-quality studies showing that regular light-to-moderate alcohol consumption offers health protection, especially pertaining to the cardiovascular and nervous systems.

Moderate alcohol consumption lowers the risk of developing cardiovascular disease and protects against future cardiovascular compromise

For example, a 2006 study published in the *Journal of the American Geriatrics Society* (302) that followed 4 410 adults over a nine-year period found that moderate alcohol consumption lowered the risk of coronary heart disease when compared with those who abstained completely.

Furthermore, a large review of the literature (303), which included eight studies involving 16 351 patients with a history of cardiovascular disease, showed that moderate alcohol consumption is associated with a lower incidence of further cardiovascular compromise and all-cause mortality. The meta-analysis asserts that maximal protection from premature mortality – which was as high as 22% – was achieved from 5–25 g of alcohol per day (0.5–2 drinks per day).

Moderate alcohol consumption may offer protection from developing diabetes

Although the cardiovascular system is often cited as a beneficiary, some studies infer that moderate alcohol consumption may offer some protection from the development of diabetes as well.

In a meta-analysis of 13 studies (304) performed at the Karolinska Institute in Sweden, researchers showed that moderate daily alcohol consumption reduces the risk of developing diabetes by up to 30%. Before getting too excited and reaching for another glass of wine, bear in mind that the study did show an aggressive U-curve, meaning that exceeding 2–3 drinks per day would actually increase the risk of developing diabetes, as well as many other diseases.

Moderate alcohol consumption boosts longevity

Yet another area of contention is the relationship between moderate alcohol consumption and lifespan. A large meta-analysis of 34 studies (305) attempted to shed light on this debate. The review, which was published in *Archives of Internal Medicine*, involved over a million participants and identified a J-shaped relationship between alcohol and total mortality in both men and women. In a nutshell, a J-shaped relationship means that low-to-moderate alcohol consumption could promote health to a degree; however, larger amounts were severely antagonistic to well-being.

Surprisingly, the study found that men were able to consume as many as four drinks per day,[5] whereas women were limited to no more than two drinks per day.[6] Furthermore, the data revealed that regular light-to-moderate alcohol consumption could lower the risk of premature mortality in men and women by as much as 17% and 18% respectively.

Light alcohol consumption may actually protect the brain in older groups

Contrary to the recently published study by researchers at Oxford, there is evidence showing that light-to-moderate alcohol consumption may actually protect the brain rather than damage it. In 2008, a team of researchers at Imperial College in London published an extensive systematic review of 23 studies (306). The meta-analysis investigated the relationship between moderate alcohol consumption and cognitive decline in persons over the age of 65. Although the authors stress that the conclusions should be met with caution, they did find that light-to-moderate alcohol consumption in early adult life offers a certain degree of protection against the development of dementia and Alzheimer's disease in our later adult years.

Light-to-moderate wine consumption may boost cognitive aptitude[7]

Not only is there evidence that light-to-moderate alcohol consumption reduces the risk of certain neurological diseases in the elderly, according to a study published in *Neurology* (307), it may provide better cognitive functioning across multiple domains when compared with complete abstinence.

Supporting these findings, a large French study (308) involving over 3 000 participants found that moderate alcohol consumption of 1–3 drinks per day is associated with higher cognitive scores[8] when compared with complete abstinence or, conversely, excessive drinking. Interestingly, the 13-year study revealed a rather unexpected twist. The researchers found an inverse association between beer consumption and cognitive performance. Essentially, beer did not provide the same benefit as wine. No explanation of why this is the case was given, but it might have to do with the wide array of phytochemicals that are found in wine, including resveratrol.

Finally, to add even more controversy to this subject, in 2015, US researchers published a study entitled "Effects of alcohol consumption on cognition and regional brain volumes among older adults" (309). The study set out to establish the relationship between mid-life and late-life alcohol consumption and regional brain volume together with cognitive functioning. Additional criteria included no history of alcohol abuse or dementia. Complex statistical models factored in both age and alcohol intake.

The results indicated that moderate alcohol consumption in late-life, but not in mid-life, is associated with better episodic memory and increased brain volume. The authors concluded that compared to late-life abstainers, moderate consumers had larger brains and better memory.

Despite all the support for light-to-moderate alcohol consumption, the evidence has not stirred health policy amendments. The debate is likely to continue, leaving the layperson confused and in need of a clearer directive.

ALCOHOL AND CHRONIC STRESS

IT'S THE END OF THE WEEK. And it's been a tough one. Relentless demands at work, insufficient sleep, challenges with interpersonal relationships, probably due to irritability and a smidgen of irrationality on my part. I've put hours and hours into work, but have an underlying uneasiness, a sense that I'm not quite on top of things.

I'm beginning to think that my biggest issue is that I feel that I'm not getting enough support from those around me. The accumulated strain of the week drives me to seek temporary respite. Perhaps a night out with friends or family and a drink or two is not just appealing, it's a necessity.

The rest is history. While the night out certainly offered a temporary escape psychologically, the next day's hangover makes any productive endeavour almost impossible. From a biological perspective, my night's drinking was nothing short of a disaster, for several reasons, which you will soon find out.

It is important to bear in mind that stress has been shown to be one of the largest influences on excess alcohol consumption, abuse and relapse behaviours (310), which is why this chapter is so important.

Stress, alcohol and the hormonal system

The hormonal system impacts every organ and cell in the body. This highly complex system comprises numerous glands that produce and secrete hormones directly into the bloodstream. Many aspects of our health and functionality are controlled through these hormonal pathways, including:

- metabolism
- energy production
- immune behaviour
- fluid balance
- growth
- cell regeneration
- development, and
- reproduction.

The hormonal system also plays an important role in enabling the body to respond to and cope with both internal and external environmental changes, and as you know, plays a central role in the management of stress.

In recent years, there has been a substantial amount of research showing that alcohol consumption, regardless of quantity, can have serious adverse effects on the components of the hormonal system, but specifically the stress axis. According to an article entitled "Effects of alcohol on the endocrine system" (311) *acute* alcohol consumption[9] results in significant increases in the circulating levels of both adrenalin and cortisol. The degree of stress hormone elevation and subsequent systemic strain appears to be dose-related, in that the higher the alcohol consumption, the greater the stress hormone spike.

The effects of chronic alcohol exposure are more complex. For example, a study published in the *International Journal of Psychophysiology* (312) showed that in heavy drinkers, cortisol levels are not just elevated in response to the immediate consumption of alcohol, but remain chronically elevated! This increase in overall cortisol levels suggests an inability to shut down the stress response[10] in the brain and body. This will leave us burnt out, exhausted, run down, emotionally and cognitively compromised, and it will have a significant impact on all areas of our life and health.

> **Warning:** Heavy alcohol consumption triggers the stress axis into overdrive to the extent that it fails to shut down!

Long periods of heavy alcohol consumption can lead to adrenal fatigue

Several studies have shown that chronic heavy alcohol consumption can also blunt the stress response, causing the adrenal glands to underproduce adrenalin and cortisol, thereby impairing coping mechanisms and negatively influencing performance (311). Consider that significant underproduction of cortisol can lead to chronic fatigue, anxiety, muscle and joint pain, and a plethora of negative biological shifts. It can even result in significant mood disturbances.

One thing is for certain, excessive alcohol consumption over prolonged periods of time does not allow us to thrive and become the best version of ourselves.

Alcohol and cortisol

In 2008, a team of German and English researchers published a study (313) on the relationship between alcohol consumption and cortisol secretion in an ageing population. A total of 3 670 men and women took part in the two-year study, during which time cortisol was measured at regular intervals throughout the day. The researchers discovered that there was a direct association between cortisol levels and the number of units of alcohol participants consumed in a week, specifically in men. For every additional unit[11] consumed, there was a corresponding rise in cortisol of 3%. So, having ten drinks in a week will increase your cortisol levels by 30% that week.

The study also showed that ongoing, heavy alcohol consumption is associated with a significant disruption in the normal daily rhythm of cortisol secretion. This daily cycle of cortisol production[12] is necessary for sleep-wake cycles. Any disturbance could create challenges, such as fatigue during the day and insomnia at night.

Even though the most reliable predictor of increased cortisol secretion and disrupted daily cortisol rhythms in men was the amount of alcohol they consumed over a week, frequent but moderate alcohol intakes appeared not to be overly impactful or disruptive.

The assertions of this study were confirmed when Dutch researchers published findings (314) on the relationship between various alcohol consumption habits and stress hormones. The Dutch study involved just under 3 000 participants with varied alcohol consumption behaviours. These included non-drinkers, moderate drinkers and heavy drinkers. As suggested in the earlier English and German study, the outcomes showed that current heavy alcohol use, rather than continual moderate alcohol consumption, was associated with greater hyperactivity of the stress axis as well as increased cardiac excitability.[13]

Alcohol's effect on women

Women have to be especially mindful of the relationship between alcohol and stress.

While it is reliably shown that men can consume alcohol moderately with minimal effect on the stress axis, the same cannot be said of women. The literature repeatedly shows that all forms of alcohol consumption – whether light, frequent, heavy or excessive – are associated with a wide array of adverse effects on a woman's stress axis. Women are therefore more likely to have:

- higher adrenalin and cortisol spikes
- a more pronounced dysregulation of the stress response, and
- greater health compromise in response to alcohol exposure, regardless of amount or frequency.

Heavy alcohol consumption results in system failure

Unlike the ongoing debate about whether or not moderate alcohol consumption offers benefits to health, the excessive consumption of alcohol and its relationship to stress is one-way traffic, even in men. The reason is partly the potential for alcohol abuse or dependence, which is a very real concern, but also the fact that alcohol consumption has a damaging effect on many of the stress-moderating centres, which will inevitably lead to systemic failure.

Here's why systemic failure is inevitable:

1. Excessive or chronic alcohol consumption damages liver function and may therefore reduce the body's ability to metabolise cortisol and other stress hormones. This leads not only to chronically elevated stress hormone profiles, but also altered hormonal function (313).

2. Prolonged or excessive alcohol consumption disrupts the functioning of the stress axis master regulator – the vagus nerve (312). This leads to an inability to shut the stress response down, resulting in prolonged elevations of cortisol and adrenalin. The net effect of protracted cortisol and adrenalin output is biological exhaustion, which leads to progressive multi-system breakdown.

3. Heavy alcohol consumption can impair the stress response within the brain, resulting in a blunted or an exaggerated effect. Neither of these responses promotes optimal functioning, performance or health in any domain.

ALCOHOL, STRESS AND GROWTH HORMONE

Stress negatively impacts all parts of our biological make-up through a variety of molecular processes, but principally through changes in our hormonal and cell signalling systems. One of the more impactful influences is a disruption in the growth hormone axis, which can be so damaging that, according to research published in *Endocrine* (315), the disruption can be seen on a genetic level.

There are very few hormones that have as broad a range of functions as growth hormone. As the name implies, growth hormone promotes growth, cell reproduction and cell regeneration. According to a 2016 article published in *Clinical Medicine Insights: Endocrinology and Diabetes* (316), the range of biological effects of growth hormone is incredible and vast. This hormone positively influences the reproductive, cardiovascular, musculoskeletal and nervous systems. It is also vital to liver, adrenal and kidney function, not to mention a wide array of other influences.

Since stress significantly impacts the growth hormone axis (317), we cannot afford to incur further compromise. In fact, all our activities and behaviours should be directed towards *optimising* this axis in order to promote stress resilience and protection.

Growth hormone levels plummet

Alcohol negatively impacts the growth hormone axis and can therefore amplify the negative effects of chronic stress in many domains. Numerous studies on both humans and animals have shown that excessive alcohol exposure[14] reduces circulating growth hormone levels. A small study by Finnish researchers (318) on the effects of heavy alcohol exposure and the hormonal system showed that three hours of heavy alcohol intake increases cortisol levels by an average of 36% the following day and has a significant effect on growth hormone secretion. The study also found that heavy alcohol consumption, even for short periods of time, reduces testosterone levels by an average of 23%.

Several animal studies have investigated the persistent effects of heavy alcohol consumption on growth hormone profiles. A study published in *Endocrinology* (319) showed that six days of heavy alcohol intake[15] resulted in genetic changes in growth hormone expression and a reduction in output by 75–90% when compared with controls. Similar results have been shown over more protracted periods. The collective results suggest that the impact of alcohol on growth hormone secretion is largely brought about by changes in the brain itself and on a genetic level, which have far-reaching consequences in the long term.

ALCOHOL AND SLEEP

Sleep is critical to our health and well-being and is profoundly impacted by acute and chronic stress. It is plausible that sleep disturbance is a contributing factor to many of the adverse health outcomes attributed to stress. Despite the fact that alcohol appears to make you drowsy, alcohol and sleep are not a good fit for a variety of reasons.

To understand the impact of alcohol on sleep behaviours, we need to have a surface knowledge of our intrinsic time-keeping system – our biorhythms.

The body's time-keeping clock is located in a region of the brain known as the suprachiasmatic nucleus. Its role is to synchronise our biological behaviour in response to external cues, such as surrounding light. These external cues are then converted into nerve or hormonal signals that ultimately affect all the body's physiological and metabolic processes, thereby allowing the body to optimise its responses to changing environmental conditions. A perfect example of this is waking up in the morning. The lighter the external environment, the more awake we are, which is why it's easy to bounce out of bed in summer, but winter is significantly more challenging!

It is important to realise that our biorhythms are dependent on the interaction of specific genes, known as **clock genes**.[16] These genes use various feedback loops and cues to maintain an almost 24-hour period of predictable cellular and biological activity.

Surprisingly, it is not only the brain (suprachiasmatic nucleus) and the clock genes that regulate our biorhythms. Various cells throughout the entire body participate in this vital process, making it a very complex process that can easily be derailed.

Numerous human and animal studies have shown that ongoing exposure to alcohol causes significant alterations in the activity of our clock genes. According to a research article by a team of German scientists (319), the consequences of clock gene failure as a direct result of alcohol consumption include:

- disrupted sleep
- abnormal body temperature
- erratic blood pressure, and
- significant changes in hormonal secretions.

None of these effects on their own, let alone collectively, would be well tolerated during periods of acute or chronic stress. It is also interesting that the article described a bidirectional relationship between clock genes and alcohol. Not only does alcohol negatively influence clock gene behaviour, abnormal clock gene behaviour results in changes in alcohol consumption habits, often leading to abuse and even dependence. Essentially, the cycle becomes self-perpetuating – the more we drink, the more we crave alcohol.

The greatest concern with alcohol's disruptive effect on our biorhythms is the fact that many of our hormones are on timers. Clock genes determine[17] the timing and quantity of many hormone secretions. The regions of the body that are principally affected include the:

- thyroid gland (thyroxine)
- adrenal glands (cortisol)
- reproductive glands (testosterone/estradiol), and
- the liver (IGF-1).

Disruptions can have far-reaching consequences in many areas of our health and functionality.

In 2004, a team of Spanish researchers published an animal study (320) looking at the effects of chronic alcohol exposure on the hormonal system over a four-week period. Not only did the scientists find that there were significant abnormalities in hormonal output, they also found that the 24-hour secretion patterns of many key hormones were severely disrupted.

It is not surprising then that alcohol abuse or dependence is linked to both the disruption of our biorhythms *and* our hormonal reactions to stress. By the same token, chronic stress is considered to be a major environmental risk factor for alcohol abuse/dependence as well as disturbed biorhythms.

The message is clear – in the interests of hormonal integrity and stress resilience, alcohol consumption should be minimal, if not altogether avoided, during periods of chronic stress.

CHAPTER SUMMARY

- There is an ongoing debate amongst scientists about whether light-to-moderate alcohol consumption is beneficial or detrimental to our health. However, all agree that the consumption of alcohol during times of stress and crisis is definitely detrimental.
- Arguments *against* light-to-moderate alcohol consumption say that it:
  - causes millions of deaths per year worldwide
  - contributes to more than 200 diseases and injury-related health conditions
  - carries the risk of abuse
  - is linked to the development of certain cancers
  - shrinks the brain and compromises the nervous system.
- Arguments *for* light-to-moderate alcohol consumption say that it:

- □ lowers the risk of developing cardiovascular disease
- □ protects against future cardiovascular compromise
- □ protects against developing diabetes
- □ promotes health and extends lifespan
- □ protects the brains of older persons against cognitive decline
- □ boosts cognitive aptitude, if in the form of wine.
- There are gender differences in terms of alcohol metabolism:
  - □ Men can consume alcohol very moderately with little effect on the stress axis.
  - □ Women do not have this advantage – any type of alcohol intake during stressful times exacerbates a woman's stress response.
- The more alcohol you consume within a week, the higher your cortisol levels.
- Heavy alcohol consumption (acute or chronic) and the stress axis:
  - □ causes significant spikes in both adrenalin and cortisol
  - □ can cause cortisol levels to remain chronically elevated
  - □ disrupts the daily rhythm of cortisol secretion
  - □ in the long term has the potential to impair the body's ability to produce the necessary amounts of cortisol and adrenalin resulting in chronic fatigue and immune disorders.
- Heavy alcohol consumption alters the functionality of numerous biological systems. For example, it:
  - □ damages the liver, reducing its ability to metabolise stress hormones
  - □ disrupts the functioning of the vagus nerve
  - □ lowers growth hormone production by as much as 75–90% due to its influence on genetic behaviours
  - □ causes significant alternations in the activity of our clock genes, impacting sleep patterns and broader hormonal balance.
- For all these reasons and the fact that stress is one of the biggest drivers in alcohol abuse behaviours, alcohol consumption should be minimal, if not altogether avoided during periods of chronic stress.

10

PUTTING IT ALL TOGETHER

The Stress Code has taken us on a journey of discovery to gain a deeper understanding of the important role that stress plays in our lives. At this stage, we know that stress enhances our abilities and potential, but only when it's sporadic and channelled appropriately. With our newly acquired knowledge, we can now differentiate between acute and chronic stress in terms of the impact they have on our health and functionality. More importantly, we know that how we perceive our circumstances as well as how we behave towards ourselves and others can reduce the negative impact of chronic stress. We now have the tools to shut down stress at will and rebuild ourselves physically and mentally, even when we feel at our weakest.

My intention in writing the book was not merely to provide an environment of resilience or a means by which you can buffer the stresses and strains that life brings. Rather, I wanted to provide a vehicle by which you can create the best version of yourself. A version that not only copes with stress, but thrives in crisis – in a way that inspires others.

Moreover, I wanted to break the archetype that stress and ageing result in a weaker physical state, reduced cognitive potential and emotional strain. Armed with the latest scientific knowledge and an understanding of how to apply it in your life, the passing years need not be associated with a regressive state – rather they can bring greater aptitudes across all health and performance domains.

Consider that in order to access your greatest potential, you would need to incorporate many, if not most, of the recommended interventions as the sum of the collective is far more effective than the influence of a single practice.

BUILDING THE PERFECT RESILIENCE MODEL

Even for the experienced and most committed health enthusiast, it may be a little challenging to coordinate all the information and integrate the interventions. To make this easier, I have provided a stress continuum chart as well as four templates to choose from, at the end of this chapter. The templates vary in their level of intensity and required commitment. Their role is to give you an indication of how all the elements can be incorporated as part of a larger whole. These templates are a great starting point, but need to be fine-tuned. Your personal preferences, experience of the interventions, budget, and the time you have available all play an important role in the construction of *your* perfect resilience plan.

To ensure success, I would like to emphasise that when you choose a template, bear in mind that it must be at a level that allows you to be consistent – especially in the long term. To thrive under stressful conditions, it is paramount that your programme is a good fit with your lifestyle.

Small or big steps – know yourself
As with any new journey, it is generally best to start slowly. Begin with a few relevant interventions and lifestyle practices in the template you choose and, much like a symphony, gradually expand your repertoire as time goes on. This protects against feeling overwhelmed and will better ensure programme adherence down the line.

While this approach may be successful for many, on the other side of the continuum there are those who thrive under very different conditions. They may prefer a comprehensive action plan reinforced by an all-encompassing structure. One of the primary attractions is that expansive routines provide an element of safety and reassurance in an environment of chronic stress, which is typically characterised by a lack of control and little or no authority over decisions.

In either instance, self-awareness and knowing your relative position on the stress chart should guide you in personalising your stress resilience action plan.

Stepping out of your comfort zone

There are many instances where progress or change is not possible without a concerted push. Often it is at our lowest points that we find the motivation to step out of our comfort zone or we find ourselves pushed out with tremendous force. To become resilient in environments or situations that are immensely stressful often requires a great deal of courage: the courage to embark on the unfamiliar and the courage to move forward when you feel at your most vulnerable. It is in these very situations that tentative measures offer little reward, whereas complete submersion in a new path almost always ensures success.

Don't let irrational fears create imaginary boundaries. Be bold.

The power of the mind

By this stage it should be obvious that changing your personal stress landscape is neither a quick fix nor a one-pill solution. The value of positive dietary practices, specific exercises, environmental awareness and supplements within an effective resilience model are beyond measure. Yet success ultimately relies on one thing and one thing alone – *a shift in mindset*.

Reframing stress as a positive experience and adopting positive attitudes and behaviours towards ourselves and others needs to be continuously emphasised and worked on throughout your stress resilience journey. Remarkably, these two vitally important features that protect us from the adverse effects of stress and enable us to use stress to our advantage require little time and *no financial expense*. But they do require repetition and practice in order to become part of our intrinsic make-up. My advice is to make personal notes and read the relevant chapters more than once to inspire movement in a forward direction.

THE STRESS CONTINUUM

Eustress/healthy stress **Acute**	**Intense stress** **3–5 weeks**	
You have flexibility of the stress response, so it's "on" at the right time and "off" when not needed. **You feel:** Energised, clear and motivated **You experience:** Better attention and focus Improved mood Greater productivity Strong immune function Faster metabolism Increased strength and power Increased endurance Improved eye sight Improved sense of smell	Anxiety High blood pressure Irregular heart beat Headaches/migraines Increased inflammation Increased sweating Skin that appears aged Sexual disorders/infertility Digestive disorders Hearing loss/ringing in ears Reduced kidney function More frequent urination Sleeplessness	
Management Stress reappraisal Pro-social behaviours Multivitamins, omega-3 fatty acids Regular exercise Bimonthly body therapy Alcohol and coffee in moderation Green tea and healthy diet Adequate sleep	**Primary management** Stress reappraisal Pro-social behaviours Breathing exercises, swimming, visceral manipulation, physical therapy, massage, yoga, meditation, music therapy, cold facial immersion **Secondary management** Omega-3 fatty acids, resveratrol, cacao, multivitamin, B-complex, ashwagandha, *Bacopa monnieri*, curcumin, green tea and magnesium Regular exercise	

Relentless stress Months or years	BURNOUT Chronic
Overproduction of cortisol Possible over-activity of the thyroid gland High susceptibility to colds and flu Increased appetite and weight gain Reflux High blood pressure Digestive issues Muscle and tendon injuries Spinal degeneration and disorders Anxiety and panic disorders Obsessive compulsive disorder Compromised learning ability Poor focus and attention Impaired memory Insomnia Cravings for sugary and fatty foods	Collapse of adrenal and thyroid function Burnout – mental and physical Difficulty getting out of bed in the morning Depression Chronic fatigue Fibromyalgia Allergies Asthma Autoimmune diseases Significant injuries Pain syndromes (lower back) Insomnia Overuse of stimulants and alcohol
Management (all carry equal weight) Reappraisal, pro-social behaviours Breathing exercises, swimming, visceral manipulation, physical therapy or massage, yoga, meditation Calming music, daily outdoor activity Omega-3 fatty acids, resveratrol, curcumin, cacao, multivitamin or B-complex, ashwagandha, *Bacopa monnieri*, *Rhodiola rosea*, curcumin, green tea Regular exercise and intermittent fasting Probiotic, magnesium, green juices, fruits and vegetables and healthy proteins	**Primary management** *Bacopa monnieri*, ashwagandha, *Rhodiola rosea*, multivitamin or B-complex, curcumin, resveratrol, omega-3 fatty acids, a broad- spectrum probiotic, magnesium Visceral manipulation **Secondary management** Yoga, meditation, music, breathing exercises, massage or physical therapy Daily outdoor activity Regular but light exercise Small frequent meals (vegetables, fruits and proteins) Limit or cut out coffee and alcohol

Consistency over time

TWO OF THE GREATEST THEMES that govern the marketing campaigns of large investment funds and financial institutions are the concepts of time and consistency – and for good reason.

In my professional experience, those who achieve the greatest results in their chosen endeavours take a long-term view and are consistent in their approach to achieving the end result.

I could give countless examples of CEOs, companies, teams or even individuals, but there is one stand-out case that embodies this philosophy. My relationship with this athlete goes back the better part of one and a half decades. Incredibly, we started working together in his early teens and I still work with him to this day.

I have to admit our initial connection was a mutual recognition that 'average' and 'mediocre' don't have a place in either of our lives. We were also somewhat outsiders. I never followed convention in any context, and when I look back, nor did he. As a junior, he barely had the support of the local tennis federation and seldom participated in the established squads or group coaching sessions. He also wasn't a fan of the physical training programmes that were popular at the time, and certainly never got caught up in fads or hype.

Even at an early age, he clearly knew where he wanted to go and what he wanted to achieve, and would spend the next fifteen years finding the best way to get there – regardless of the challenges or sacrifices. It certainly hasn't been an easy road for him. There have been several hurdles in the form of injuries.

What many people don't realise is that two things typically accompany significant injuries in a high-precision, individual sport like tennis. The first is compensation in movement patterns and technique, which is extremely hard to overcome. This predisposes the player to further injury, but more concerning, it manifests in erratic performances. The second is a blow to confidence, largely triggered by the poor results following an injury.

There have been two significant injury setbacks that unfolded for him in recent years. Consider that very few injuries in tennis result from a single trauma. Most are insidious by nature and develop progressively. His first injury was just that, a progressive increase in pain in his left knee that escalated over a period of time. By early 2014, playing became challenging and competing at a high level near impossible. Up to this point, there had been steady progress in his ranking, maintaining a consistent spot in the top 20. However, his knee injury limited his speed around the court and impacted his most powerful weapon – his serve.

In April 2014, I decided to join the player for the European leg of the tour, which started in Madrid and ended at Wimbledon. The first three weeks of treatment and physical management were tough for a number of reasons, the primary one being the fact that he was competing during the treatment process.

Initially, progress was predictably slow and results from the first few tournaments average at best. Yet this did not faze him. He always looked to the future and applied his greatest strengths to the recovery process – discipline and a stringent work ethic.

At the end of every day, he would reflect, looking for more areas or aspects he could improve on. His ethos during this time was: what more do I need to do to improve? This is in stark contrast to the general trend in society, where impatience and a fixation on the here and now completely predominate.

The time we spent together was heavily invested in rehabilitating the injured area, improving health practices (vagal stimulation, diet, training, recovery techniques), as well as working on physical weaknesses, including movement.

By the end of the three-month period, the knee injury had fully resolved, movement was at an all-time high, as were his results and even his ranking. I recall sitting in the player box on Centre Court at Wimbledon thinking, what a journey. Yet he was still to realise the greatest benefit from all his effort and hard work.

Just over a year later, he achieved a lifetime goal – breaking into the top 10 in the ATP rankings after beating a long-time adversary – incidentally, the player who had beaten him at Wimbledon the previous year – to get into the quarter-finals of the US Open.

So many people chase the quick fix at the expense of true success. The lesson one can take away from this athlete's story is that he based his success on his intrinsic faith in the outcome, his strong desire to improve, his commitment and consistency and, most importantly, his patience. I have to mention that throughout this period his support from his wife and the rest of the team was incredible, highlighting the value of social bonds during crisis.

However, this was only the first of the major setbacks. The second proved to be a far greater test of character than the first, and almost ended his career.

Towards the end of 2016, he sustained a significant hip injury while competing in Europe. In many instances, an injury of this nature would mean surgery and almost a year off, with no guarantees of ever returning to full fitness. After much thought and consulting with experts around the world, he decided to return to South Africa and receive treatment for as long as it took.

I freed up several hours a day, six days a week. I considered all the elements in the recovery process, including diet to support healing, therapeutic exercise to support treatment, nutritional supplements to reduce inflammation and even a strategic model for his re-entry into tennis. The fragility and instability of the affected region meant that rehabilitation had to be comprehensive and methodical. Every body segment had to be carefully considered in light of its relationship to the injured area. Moreover, controlling inflammation was the cornerstone of treatment. The vagus nerve was central to the process. Two-hour treatment sessions were the norm.

Throughout the course of treatment, he was totally composed, never anxious and incredibly positive. Like two years earlier, his commitment and trust in the process were unwavering and his work ethic exemplary. The perfect example of how reframing stress can positively influence outcomes.

Within ten days, his pain had decreased enough to start hitting a few balls. His return to the tennis court was extremely conservative, starting with hitting balls against a practice wall for 30 minutes. He did this several times. I have to say that seeing an athlete of this calibre return to basics is both humbling and inspiring! By the end of three weeks, he had made significant progress, so much so that he was training normally and practising conservatively.

When he returned to competitive tennis, his results were slow at first, but in August of 2017 he stamped his authority on the sport by reaching the final of the US Open and smashing into the top 10 rankings once again. But this was only the beginning. Ten months later at the 2018 Wimbledon Championships he became a household name through a courageous and inspiring journey to the final. He staged one of the most impressive comebacks in tennis history against Roger Federer, from being match point down to win in the quarter-finals. If that wasn't enough, his mental and physical toughness helped him secure a win in a gruelling six and a half hour semi-final. It became apparent that his challenges had made him stronger, wiser and more focused than ever before. This, together with a great supportive team – wife, trainer, physio, coaches and friends – have propelled him into the top five in the world rankings with no signs of slowing down.

The central theme in these experiences is that for the interventions and tools provided in this book to be successful, you have to commit yourself totally to the process. Moreover, you need to be consistent in your efforts as well as continue to find ways to constantly improve. Finally, success takes time. Be patient and always look forward, like the athlete – *it will be well worth it.*

STRESS RESILIENCE TEMPLATES

THE BASIC APPROACH	Monday	Tuesday	Wednesday
Weekly focus points	Stress reappraisal, engage in more pro-social behaviours, endeavour to reduce stress footprint		
Diet and lifestyle	Include: Green tea, cacao/cocoa-rich foods, turmeric + black pepper, dark berries		
	Limit or cut out: Processed sugar, alcohol (max 1–2 units per day), coffee (1–2 per day)		
Exercise/ activity	Aerobic exercise (walk, run, cycle, swim) 20–60 min		Yoga 45–90 min
Therapies			
Environment Check UV radiation to ensure safe sun practices		10–20 min outdoors between 10 am and 2 pm	
Morning supplements	Omega-3 fatty acid, multivitamin, Ashwagandha	Omega-3 fatty acid, multivitamin, Ashwagandha	Omega-3 fatty acid, multivitamin, Ashwagandha
Afternoon supplement	Ashwagandha	Ashwagandha	Ashwagandha
Before bed	5–12 min breathing exercises	Meditation practice of choice or 30–45 min of relaxing music	5–12 min breathing exercises
Additional strategies			

Thursday	Friday	Saturday	Sunday
Stress reappraisal, engage in more pro-social behaviours, endeavour to reduce stress footprint			
Include: Green tea, cacao/cocoa-rich foods, turmeric + black pepper, dark berries			
Limit or cut out: Processed sugar, alcohol (max 1–2 units per day), coffee (1–2 per day)			
	Weight training: Circuit format/ body weight exercises		
	Visceral manipulation or massage or physical therapy		
10–20 min outdoors between 10 am and 2 pm		10–20 min outdoors between 10 am and 2 pm	
Omega-3 fatty acid, multivitamin, Ashwagandha	Omega-3 fatty acid, multivitamin, Ashwagandha	Omega-3 fatty acid, multivitamin, Ashwagandha	Omega-3 fatty acid, multivitamin, Ashwagandha
Ashwagandha	Ashwagandha	Ashwagandha	Ashwagandha
Meditation practice of choice or 30–45 min of relaxing music		5–12 min breathing exercises	Meditation practice of choice or 30–45 min of relaxing music
			Intermittent fast (14–16 hours)

THE ENTHUSIASTIC MODERATE	Monday	Tuesday	Wednesday
Weekly focus points	Stress reappraisal, engage in more pro-social behaviours, endeavour to reduce stress footprint		
Diet and lifestyle	Include: Green tea, cacao/cocoa-rich foods, turmeric + black pepper, dark berries		
	Limit or cut out: Processed sugar, alcohol (max 1–2 units per day), coffee (1–2 per day)		
Exercise/ activity	Yoga 45–90 min		Swimming: Easy with varied strokes for 15–30 min OR another form of aerobic exercise for >30 min
Therapies	Massage or therapy of choice for 30–60 min		
Environment Check UV radiation to ensure safe sun practices	10–20 min outdoors between 10 am and 2 pm	10–20 min outdoors between 10 am and 2 pm	
Morning supplements	Omega-3 fatty acid, multivitamin, *Rhodiola rosea*, Ashwagandha	Omega-3 fatty acid, multivitamin, *Rhodiola rosea*, Ashwagandha	Omega-3 fatty acid, multivitamin, *Rhodiola rosea*, Ashwagandha
Afternoon supplements	Ashwagandha, *Rhodiola rosea*	Ashwagandha, *Rhodiola rosea*	Ashwagandha, *Rhodiola rosea*
Before bed		Meditation practice of choice or 30–45 min of relaxing music	5–12 min breathing exercises
Additional strategies			

Thursday	Friday	Saturday	Sunday
Stress reappraisal, engage in more pro-social behaviours, endeavour to reduce stress footprint			
Include: Green tea, cacao/cocoa-rich foods, turmeric + black pepper, dark berries			
Limit or cut out: Processed sugar, alcohol (max 1–2 units per day), coffee (1–2 per day)			
	Weight training: Circuit format/ body weight exercises		
	Visceral manipulation or physical therapy		
10–20 min outdoors between 10 am and 2 pm	10–20 min outdoors between 10 am and 2 pm		
Omega-3 fatty acid, multivitamin, *Rhodiola rosea*, Ashwagandha	Omega-3 fatty acid, multivitamin, *Rhodiola rosea*, Ashwagandha	Omega-3 fatty acid, multivitamin, *Rhodiola rosea*, Ashwagandha	Omega-3 fatty acid, multivitamin, *Rhodiola rosea*, Ashwagandha
Ashwagandha, *Rhodiola rosea*	Ashwagandha, *Rhodiola rosea*	Ashwagandha, *Rhodiola rosea*	Ashwagandha, *Rhodiola rosea*
Meditation practice of choice or 30–45 min of relaxing music		5–12 min breathing exercises	Meditation practice of choice or 30–45 min of relaxing music
			Intermittent fast (14–16 hours)

THE ALL-IN	Monday	Tuesday	Wednesday
Weekly focus points	Stress reappraisal, engage in more pro-social behaviours, endeavour to reduce stress footprint		
Diet and lifestyle	Include: Green tea, cacao/cocoa-rich foods, dark berries		
	Limit or cut out: Processed sugar, alcohol (max 1–2 units per day), coffee (1 per day)		
Exercise/ activity	Yoga 45–90 min	Aerobic exercise in an interval fashion (subject to fitness level and equipment availability)	Swimming: Easy with varied strokes for 15–30 min
Therapies	Massage or therapy of choice for 30 min		
Environment Check UV radiation to ensure safe sun practices	10–20 min outdoors between 10 am and 2 pm	10–20 min outdoors between 10 am and 2 pm	
Morning supplements	Omega-3 fatty acid, multivitamin, *Rhodiola rosea*, Ashwagandha, *Bacopa monnieri*, curcumin, resveratrol	Omega-3 fatty acid, multivitamin, *Rhodiola rosea*, Ashwagandha, *Bacopa monnieri*, curcumin, resveratrol	Omega-3 fatty acid, multivitamin, *Rhodiola rosea*, Ashwagandha, *Bacopa monnieri*, curcumin, resveratrol
Afternoon supplements	Ashwagandha, *Rhodiola rosea*, magnesium	Ashwagandha, *Rhodiola rosea*, magnesium	Ashwagandha, *Rhodiola rosea*, magnesium
Before bed	5–12 min breathing exercises	Meditation practice of choice or 30–45 min of relaxing music	5–12 min breathing exercises
Additional strategies	Optional: Weight training 30–60 minutes		Optional: Weight training 30–60 minutes

Thursday	Friday	Saturday	Sunday
Stress reappraisal, engage in more pro-social behaviours, endeavour to reduce stress footprint			
Include: Green tea, cacao/cocoa-rich foods, dark berries			
Limit or cut out: Processed sugar, alcohol (max 1–2 units per day), coffee (1 per day)			
Yoga 45–90 min	Weight training: Circuit format/ body weight exercises		Optional: >30 minutes aerobic exercise (easy)
	Visceral manipulation or physical therapy		
10–20 min outdoors between 10 am and 2 pm	10–20 min outdoors between 10 am and 2 pm		
Omega-3 fatty acid, multivitamin, *Rhodiola rosea*, Ashwagandha, *Bacopa monnieri*, curcumin, resveratrol	Omega-3 fatty acid, multivitamin, *Rhodiola rosea*, Ashwagandha, *Bacopa monnieri*, curcumin, resveratrol	Omega-3 fatty acid, multivitamin, *Rhodiola rosea*, Ashwagandha, *Bacopa monnieri*, curcumin, resveratrol	Omega-3 fatty acid, multivitamin, *Rhodiola rosea*, Ashwagandha, *Bacopa monnieri*, curcumin, resveratrol
Ashwagandha, *Rhodiola rosea*, magnesium	Ashwagandha, *Rhodiola rosea*, magnesium	Ashwagandha, *Rhodiola rosea*, magnesium	Ashwagandha, *Rhodiola rosea*, magnesium
Meditation practice of choice or 30–45 min of relaxing music		5–12 min breathing exercises	Meditation practice of choice or 30–45 min of relaxing music
			Intermittent fast (14–16 hours)

TO THE EXTREME	Monday	Tuesday	Wednesday
Weekly focus points	Stress reappraisal, engage in more pro-social behaviours, endeavour to reduce stress footprint		
Diet and lifestyle	Include: Green tea (1–3 cups per day), cacao/cocoa-rich foods, dark berries, green juice, fermented foods or probiotic		
	Limit or cut out: Processed sugar, wheat, barley, rye, alcohol (max 1–2 units per day), coffee (1 per day), limit heavily processed dairy products		
Exercise/ activity	Yoga 45–90 min	Aerobic exercise in an interval fashion (subject to fitness level and equipment availability)	Yoga 45–90 min
Therapies	Massage or therapy of choice		
Environment Check UV radiation to ensure safe sun practices	10–20 min outdoors between 10 am and 2 pm	10–20 min outdoors between 10 am and 2 pm	
Morning supplements	Omega-3 fatty acid, multivitamin, Rhodiola rosea, Ashwagandha, Bacopa monnieri, curcumin, resveratrol	Omega-3 fatty acid, multivitamin, Rhodiola rosea, Ashwagandha, Bacopa monnieri, curcumin, resveratrol	Omega-3 fatty acid, multivitamin, Rhodiola rosea, Ashwagandha, Bacopa monnieri, curcumin, resveratrol
Afternoon supplements	Ashwagandha, Rhodiola rosea, Bacopa monnieri, magnesium	Ashwagandha, Rhodiola rosea, Bacopa monnieri, magnesium	Ashwagandha, Rhodiola rosea, Bacopa monnieri, magnesium
Before bed	5–12 min breathing exercises	Meditation practice of choice or 30–45 min of relaxing music	5–12 min breathing exercises
Additional strategies			

Thursday	Friday	Saturday	Sunday
Stress reappraisal, engage in more pro-social behaviours, endeavour to reduce stress footprint			
Include: Green tea (1–3 cups per day), cacao/cocoa-rich foods, dark berries, green juice, fermented foods or probiotic			
Limit or cut out: Processed sugar, wheat, barley, rye, alcohol (max 1–2 units per day), coffee (1 per day), limit heavily processed dairy products			
Weight training: Circuit format/ body weight exercises	Aerobic exercise in a continuous fashion for 30–60 minutes (walking, running, cycling, hiking, swimming)		Swimming: Easy with varied strokes for 25–40 min
	Visceral manipulation or physical therapy		
10–20 min outdoors between 10 am and 2 pm	10–20 min outdoors between 10 am and 2 pm		10–20 min outdoors between 10 am and 2 pm
Omega-3 fatty acid, multivitamin, *Rhodiola rosea*, Ashwagandha, *Bacopa monnieri*, curcumin, resveratrol	Omega-3 fatty acid, multivitamin, *Rhodiola rosea*, Ashwagandha, *Bacopa monnieri*, curcumin, resveratrol	Omega-3 fatty acid, multivitamin, *Rhodiola rosea*, Ashwagandha, *Bacopa monnieri*, curcumin, resveratrol	Omega-3 fatty acid, multivitamin, *Rhodiola rosea*, Ashwagandha, *Bacopa monnieri*, curcumin, resveratrol
Ashwagandha, *Rhodiola rosea*, *Bacopa monnieri*, magnesium	Ashwagandha, *Rhodiola rosea*, *Bacopa monnieri*, magnesium	Ashwagandha, *Rhodiola rosea*, *Bacopa monnieri*, magnesium	Ashwagandha, *Rhodiola rosea*, *Bacopa monnieri*, magnesium
Meditation practice of choice or 30–45 min of relaxing music		5–12 min breathing exercises	Meditation practice of choice or 30–45 min of relaxing music
			Don't combine fasting with demanding exercise protocols

TEMPLATE FOR YOUR OWN STRESS RESILIENCE PROGRAMME

YOUR PERSONAL PROGRAMME	Monday	Tuesday	Wednesday
Weekly focus points	Stress reappraisal, engage in more pro-social behaviours, endeavour to reduce stress footprint		
My diet and lifestyle commitments			
Exercise/ activity			
Therapies			
Environment Check UV radiation to ensure safe sun practices			
Morning supplements			
Afternoon supplements			
Before bed			
Additional strategies			

Thursday	Friday	Saturday	Sunday
Stress reappraisal, engage in more pro-social behaviours, endeavour to reduce stress footprint			

NOTES

Chapter 1 Introduction

1. My protocol included exercising outdoors and consuming extra fluids to combat dehydration. If I could, I would book a massage and spend 15–20 minutes in a sauna. When jet-lagged, avoid alcohol and take an antioxidant formulation as well as melatonin.
2. A hormone triggered by stress that increases heart rate and respiration, and prepares the muscles for activity.
3. A hormone triggered by stress that releases glucose into the bloodstream, metabolises fats, proteins and carbohydrates, and suppresses the immune system.
4. A system of complementary medicine in which a variety of medical disorders are treated through manipulation of the skeletal, fascial, muscular, nervous, vascular and visceral systems.

Chapter 2 The Science of Stress

1. Endocrine (hormonal), nervous, cardiovascular, digestive, immune, respiratory and reproductive.
2. Chromosomes are the carriers of deoxyribonucleic acid (DNA).
3. Longer telomeres are associated with better health.
4. An individual's mental and emotional state in the context of his or her social environment.
5. Testing for systemic inflammation involves looking at C-reactive protein levels in the body.
6. Highly unstable and damaging molecules.
7. Oxidative stress is an imbalance between the production of harmful free radicals and the ability of the body to counteract or neutralise their effects through antioxidants.

8. Cardiovascular, immune, hormonal and nervous.
9. The amygdala are two areas in the brain – one in each hemisphere – that play a primary role in decision-making and memory of emotional responses, especially fear.
10. Also known as epinephrine.
11. Molecules that reduce our perception of pain.
12. Conditions in which our immune system attacks our cells and tissues, such as multiple sclerosis and Type 1 diabetes mellitus.
13. The hormone that lowers sugar levels in the bloodstream.
14. The hormone that promotes youth and vitality.
15. The spontaneous peristaltic movements of the stomach that aid in digestion and moving food through the stomach.
16. The weight in kilograms divided by the square of the height in metres.
17. Prefrontal cortex, insular cortex and anterior cingulate.
18. Hippocampus and amygdala.
19. A blank cell that can develop into a variety of different cells.
20. The hippocampus is largely responsible for emotions and memory and is a prominent feature in emotional and behavioural disorders.

Chapter 3 Stress in the Workplace
1. See www.stress.org.
2. An employee's rank or position within the organisation.
3. See http://www.hse.gov.uk.
4. This is the same meta-study used to support data presented in *Chapter 2 The Science of Stress*.

Chapter 4 Cracking the Stress Code
1. Power, team sports and endurance athletes.
2. Swimming, athletics, tennis and soccer.
3. Curling, golf and cricket.
4. Ice baths, contrast showers.
5. Elevated growth hormone and reduced cortisol.

Chapter 5 Step 1: Change your Perception of Stress
1. The heart pumped more blood to the brain and body.
2. Also known as the hypothalamic-pituitary-adrenal (HPA) axis, the stress axis refers to the interactions between the nervous system and the endocrine system during the stress response.
3. Graduate Record Examination, an extremely stringent test that applicants must pass in

order to study at Harvard.

4. A one- to two-year basic military training in one of the armed forces was compulsory in South Africa at that time.

Chapter 6 Step 2: Change your Behaviour

1. A small region in the centre of the brain that controls the involuntary nervous system and hormone secretion by the pituitary gland. The hypothalamus uses these two channels to regulate vital processes, such as blood pressure, thirst, hunger, sleep and wakefulness cycles, and body temperature.
2. Known as the master gland, this pea-sized gland at the base of the brain controls all other endocrine glands. It also controls biological growth and development.
3. Specifically of the OXTR gene.
4. These are the AA/AG genotypes.
5. A division of the involuntary nervous system that restores organ functionality and hormonal balance, and has an overall calming effect.
6. The vagus nerve is covered in more detail in *Chapter 7 Step 3: Shut it Down.*
7. Helping strangers or friends in need, charity, showing empathy, and so on.
8. The experience of feeling or emotion.
9. A well-validated measure of mental health.

Chapter 7 Step 3: Shut it Down

1. Impaired or abnormal regulation.
2. This is done by sending regular electrical impulses to the vagus nerves via an implanted electrode or a handheld device.
3. This can be measured by an electrocardiogram (ECG).
4. A chemical messenger.
5. A type of white blood cell.
6. Tumour Necrosis Factor (TNF) is a protein that promotes inflammation.
7. Chronic inflammation of the bowel.
8. Stress disrupts the movement of organs and glands and this change causes an alarm reaction and more stress.
9. Commonly referred to as the 'happiness hormone'.
10. Neurotransmitters are chemical agents that enable the transfer of impulses from neuron to neuron.
11. Commonly referred to as the 'thinking hormone'.
12. These are typically associated with meditation, yoga and heart rate variability biofeedback.
13. Notably, the aortic arch and the carotid sinus.
14. Baroreceptors and the mechanoreceptors in the smooth muscle of the lung and vagal

sub-diaphragmatic branches.

15. For those who don't play tennis, tennis shoes are vastly different from normal training shoes in many respects, including grip, ankle support and weight.

16. I did find a way to treat it.

17. In relation to the body, many factors contributing to a healthy outcome is always a good thing.

18. Cold water facial immersion is discussed in more detail in the next section.

19. Lower resting heart rate.

20. Cranial sacral therapy is a gentle, hands-on method of evaluating and enhancing the functioning of a craniosacral system, comprising the membranes and cerebrospinal fluid that surround and protect the brain and spinal cord.

21. Emotional Freedom Technique (EFT) is self-help therapy that draws on various theories of alternative health modalities, including acupuncture, neurolinguistic programming, energy medicine, and Thought Field Therapy (TFT). During a typical EFT session, the person will focus on a specific emotional or physical issue while tapping on specific points along the body's energy meridians.

22. Subtle variances in heart rate between beats.

23. 7- to 9-year-olds.

24. Depression was measured according to the Hamilton Depression Rating scale.

25. From Harvard Medical School, Georgetown University Medical Center, Boston University School of Medicine, Rush University Medical Center and Massachusetts General Hospital.

26. A condition characterised by six or more months of chronic, exaggerated worry and tension, which is either unfounded or much more severe than the normal anxiety most people experience.

27. This is a standard experimental technique for inducing a stress response, in which participants are asked on short notice to give a speech in front of an audience. They are also given other anxiety-inducing instructions.

28. Adrenocorticotropic hormone, which is the hormone that signals the adrenal glands to produce cortisol.

29. The Trier Social Stress Test.

30. The structure or form of an object.

31. A sophisticated neuro-imaging analysis technique that provides a clear view of focal differences in the brain's anatomy.

32. A cell that supports and insulates brain cells.

33. A family of proteins that promotes the survival, development and function of nerve cells.

34. Zen meditation focuses on the breath and staying in the present moment.

35. Neuroplasticity refers to the brain's innate ability to change, remodel and reorganise for the purpose of greater adaptability to new situations.

36. Prefrontal cortex.

37. A keen awareness and attention to our thoughts and feelings in the present moment.

38. Increased activity.
39. A key molecule that controls the expression of inflammation-related genes.
40. Clinical groups are composed of participants involved in a specific healthcare trial.
41. Developed by Professor Jon Kabat-Zinn at the University of Massachusetts.
42. The supplementary motor area, pre-supplementary cortex, cingulate cortex, insular cortex, frontal gyrus and premotor cortex.
43. Professor Tang is an expert in the field of neuroscience and by 2018 had published eight books and more than 290 peer-reviewed articles.
44. Premotor cortex, parts of the prefrontal cortex and anterior/mid cingulate cortex.
45. This is covered in *Step 2: Change your Behaviour.*
46. How hard the athletes thought they were pushing themselves.
47. Attention, focus and euphoria chemicals.
48. Positron-Emission Tomography.
49. Insula, anterior cingulate cortex, orbitofrontal cortex and nucleus accumbens.
50. Various styles of dance music characterised by electronic sounds and a high-energy, rhythmic beat.
51. Study controls, the nature of stress stimulus, sample size.
52. A biomarker of activity in the sympathetic nervous system.
53. Heart rate variability.
54. Elevated allostatic load.
55. Elevated adrenalin and noradrenalin.
56. Cytokines.
57. A self-reported sleep questionnaire that assesses sleep quality over a one-month period. Overall scores range from 0 to 21. Lower scores denote healthier sleep quality.
58. Chinese instrumental music, classical music, nature sounds.
59. Sleep quality is defined by tiredness on waking and throughout the day, feeling rested and restored on waking, and the number of awakenings experienced in the night.
60. These brain waves are involved in conscious thought and logical thinking, and have a strong arousal effect.
61. Viruses, yeasts, bacteria.
62. A protein produced by blood plasma cells to counteract the damaging effects of microorganisms and foreign bodies (antigens).
63. Nose, eyes, lungs, genital area.
64. Glucocorticoid receptor resistance.
65. Music therapy is the clinical and evidence-based use of music interventions to accomplish individualised goals within a therapeutic relationship with an accredited professional who has completed an approved music therapy programme.
66. The role of growth hormone is discussed in *Step 4: Rebuild and Repair.*
67. A Mediterranean diet.
68. Meat, butter, cream, processed oils – essentially a Western diet.
69. Olive oil, seeds, nuts, fish oils.

70. A typical Western diet.
71. Saturated fat formed 20% of the caloric intake.
72. Low-density lipoprotein, commonly known as the 'bad' cholesterol.

Chapter 8 Step 4: Rebuild and Repair

1 Nerve growth factor, brain-derived neurotrophic factor (BDNF), neurotrophin 3 and neurotrophin 4.
2. The formation of new brain cells.
3. BDNF does this by binding with synapses and increasing the flow of ions.
4. Sprints interchanged with slow jogging.
5. Organelles found inside every cell that are responsible for energy production.
6. See interval options in the section on BDNF.
7. There is a higher prevalence of autoimmune, psychiatric and cardiovascular diseases during the winter months.
8. The outer layer of the skin.
9. Found in morning sun rays.
10. Serotonin is a neurotransmitter that plays an important role in cognition (memory, learning), emotional integrity, social interactions, sleep, appetite and digestion.
11. Early in the 20th century, vitamins were known as 'vital amines' because they were incorrectly thought to contain proteins. They are still considered vital for life, however.
12. A vitamin B9 and B12 deficiency can impair the natural liberation process that occurs through sun exposure. The liberation process involves nitrite and nitrate reserves in the skin, which need to be converted. B vitamins facilitate this. The role of B vitamins is discussed in the *Multivitamins* section.
13. FOXo3 and Sirtuins.
14. High-density lipoprotein cholesterol – the 'good' cholesterol.
15. Hormonal and metabolic, for example.
16. No added sugar, artificial sweeteners or milk.
17. For example, those with diabetes, adrenal fatigue, a renal disorder or an eating disorder.
18. The animal equivalent of cortisol.
19. Examples of combative sports are wrestling, boxing and the martial arts.
20. Substances that mimic other substances.
21. FOXo3 and Sirtuins.
22. The natural, regulated, destructive mechanism of the cell that disassembles unnecessary or dysfunctional components.
23. The part of a person's life in which they are in general good health.
24. Compounds in plant pigments that are powerful anti-oxidants.
25. A member of the ginger plant family.
26. Done on living organisms.
27. Responsible for our emotional make-up, behaviour and motivation.

28. The key regions of the brain responsible for memory, attention, decision-making, planning and a host of other executive skills.
29. An excitatory neurochemical found in the brain, which is responsible for sending signals between nerve cells. It plays an important functional role in learning and memory.
30. Of which curcumin is a member.
31. The clumping together of platelets, which is a necessary part of the clotting process triggered by injuries.
32. The region of the brain most affected by stress and cortisol.
33. A protein that is involved in several physiological processes, including lowered inflammation, improved insulin sensitivity, and biological processes that ensure cells remain youthful and robust.
34. Plant chemicals.
35. Refers to the natural 24-hour cycle of biological processes.
36. Their combined effect is greater than the sum of their parts.
37. Dietary choices, lifestyle behaviours and exercise habits.
38. Pumping out too much adrenalin and cortisol.
39. The area of the brain responsible for focus, planning, attention and short-term memory.
40. Stress hormones.
41. Only the DHA component.
42. For example autoimmune diseases, cancers and chronic pain.
43. For example atherosclerosis, allergies, asthma, depression.
44. One of the best ways to eliminate mercury is to sweat it out, by exercising or having a sauna.
45. Oils need to be refrigerated and protected from light.
46. Plant-derived, from seeds and nuts.
47. Chronic stress, environmental pollution, lack of sunlight, a corrupted food chain, poor food choices and an over-abundance of food additives.
48. Pyridoxine, pyridoxal, pyridoxamine.
49. Folate/folic acid.
50. Cobolamin.
51. Amino acids are the building blocks of proteins.
52. A circulatory disorder that causes narrowing of blood vessels that supply blood to the body.
53. A disease related to compromised circulation in the brain.
54. Parietal cells.
55. Longer than a year.
56. Anyone familiar with this claustrophobic procedure will understand why some of the subjects declined to undergo the scanning process.
57. For example, confusion and depression.
58. See *Chapter 3 Stress in the Workplace*.
59. The same is true for dopamine and noradrenalin.

60. Cells found in several parts of the intestine, which produce serotonin.
61. Promote synthesis and regeneration.
62. Serotonin, melatonin, dopamine, noradrenalin, adrenalin.
63. Variations.
64. Thiamine.
65. There are several health implications attributed to excess consumption of vitamin A, which are beyond the scope of this book.
66. Capsules, tablets and liquids.
67. Micrograms.
68. Compounds found in multivitamins and minerals.
69. Vitamins B9 and B12 have intertwined mechanisms.
70. Used to reduce stomach acid.
71. Often prescribed to treat high cholesterol and other medical conditions.
72. Due to increased histamine production.
73. Especially tetracyline.
74. Specifically B6, B9 and B12.
75. Norwegian Vitamin Trial and Western Norway B Vitamin Intervention Trial.
76. The most prevalent form of cancer.
77. Men who did not take vitamins B6 and B12.
78. Traditional Indian healthcare system based on balance in all body systems. Ayurveda uses diet, herbal remedies and yogic breathing as treatment modalities.
79. Cell receptors are specific proteins on the outside or inside of cells, to which various molecules such as hormones, neurotransmitters and antibodies may become bound, thereby influencing the cell's behaviour and function.
80. Hsp70.
81. FOXo3.
82. Nitric oxide.
83. c-Jun N-terminal kinases.
84. By increasing the number of free radicals.
85. JNK.
86. The architecture of cells that is visible at higher magnifications.
87. 400 mg in total per day.
88. Granulated powders and extracts.
89. Includes tomatoes, potatoes and eggplant.
90. Ashwagandha's botanical name.
91. Protein fragments that pack together between the neurons in the brain.
92. Conditions or symptoms that occur at the same time.
93. This was covered at the beginning of *Chapter 7 Step 3: Shut it Down*.
94. Toxic substances produced as part of the alcohol fermentation process that are responsible for much of the hangover.
95. Specifically acetylcholine.

96. The thymus gland is a very important organ that is largely responsible for immune function and regulation, specifically during our childhood years.
97. Meat, cold water fish, olive oil, avocado, full cream dairy products.
98. Catechins are found in green tea and cacao.
99. Polyphenols are compounds found in plants that greatly benefit the human body and help fight disease.
100. Biologically active compounds found in plants.
101. Vascular endothelial cells.
102. The effects of nitric oxide on the cardiovascular system were discussed in the *Go outdoors* section.
103. One of the largest studies conducted on stress.
104. 35 to 40 hours per week.
105. Two cups.
106. Striatum, hippocampus and hypothalamus.
107. Reduced activity in the sympathomedullary pathway.
108. Corticosterone.
109. Found in black tea, energy drinks and coffee.
110. A substance ingested primarily for its effects on the brain.
111. Insomnia, infertility, depression, anxiety.
112. Equal to four to five cups of coffee per day.
113. 3.5 mg of caffeine per kilogram of body weight.
114. According to the World Health Organization, the top six causes of mortality globally were heart disease, stroke, lower respiratory infections, chronic obstructive pulmonary disease, certain cancers and diabetes.
115. See the *Go outdoors* section for more information on the benefits of nitric oxide release.
116. Kale, broccoli, asparagus, blueberries, blackberries, green tea, dark cherries.
117. One of the principal constituents of cacao.
118. Reduce the effect of.
119. The stress hormones were scaled to the circumstances.
120. Lower stress hormone output in response to stress simulations.
121. Cortisol and adrenalin (epinephrine).
122. Intrinsic brain hormones adrenocorticotropic hormone (ACTH) and norepinephrine.
123. NF-κB.
124. IL-1B, IL-6.
125. I use the terms cacao and cocoa interchangeably from here on, with the obvious understanding that cacao has many more benefits because it is not processed.
126. BDNF promotes the development of new brain cells as well as the growth and survival of existing brain cells.
127. Angiogenesis.
128. None of whom were diabetic.
129. This refers to isolated cocoa flavanols.

130. For those with a nut sensitivity, replace the nut butter with a banana, reduce the dates to three and cut out the walnuts.
131. Carcinogens are substances that might cause cancer in living tissues.

Chapter 9 Alcohol

1. About two drinks.
2. Shrinkage, grey-matter density and white-matter characteristics.
3. This equates to about 15 double shots of pure spirit, such as whiskey or vodka.
4. 14–21 units per week.
5. There is cheering at this point when I give my talks.
6. Then the women in the audience sigh!
7. Sorry, guys, this doesn't apply to beer!
8. In testing memory and logic.
9. Copious amounts of alcohol in a single sitting, also referred to as binge drinking.
10. HPA dysregulation.
11. 10 ml of pure alcohol.
12. Cortisol's daily rhythm is described in more detail in the section on *Meditation* in *Chapter 7 Step 3: Shut it down.*
13. Elevated heart rate.
14. In a single intake or over a period of time.
15. 5% of dietary calories.
16. Period, Clock, Bmal1 and Cryptochrome.
17. Either directly or indirectly.

REFERENCES

1. Raposa, E.B., Laws, H.B., Ansell, E.B. "Prosocial behavior mitigates the negative effects of stress in everyday life." *Clinical Psychological Science* 4.4 (2016):691–98.
2. Richardson, S., et al. "Meta-analysis of perceived stress and its association with incident coronary heart disease." *The American Journal of Cardiology* 110.12 (2012):1711–16. PMC. Web. 7 Aug. 2017.
3. Goh, J., et al. "Workplace stressors & health outcomes: health policy for the workplace." *Behavioral Science & Policy* 1.1 (2015):43–52.
4. World Health Organization, Geneva. "WHO methods and data sources for global burden of disease estimates 2000–2011." Geneva: Department of Health Statistics and Information Systems (2013).
5. Kivimäki, M., et al. "Long working hours and risk of coronary heart disease and stroke: a systematic review and meta-analysis of published and unpublished data for 603 838 individuals." *The Lancet* 386.10005 (2015):1739–46.
6. Epel, E.S., Blackburn E.H., et al. "Accelerated telomere shortening in response to life stress." *Proceedings of the National Academy of Sciences of the United States of America* 101.49 (2004):17312–5.
7. "The Nobel Prize in Physiology or Medicine 2009". Nobelprize.org. Nobel Media AB 2014. Web. 14 May 2018. http://www.nobelprize.org/nobel_prizes/medicine/laureates/2009/
8. Kiecolt-Glaser, J.K., et al. "Childhood adversity heightens the impact of later-life caregiving stress on telomere length and inflammation." *Psychosomatic Medicine* 73.1 (2011):16–22.
9. Pace, T.W., Mletzko, T.C., Alagbe, O., Musselman, D.L., et al. "Increased stress-induced inflammatory responses in male patients with major depression and increased early life stress." *American Journal of Psychiatry* 163.9 (2006):1630–33.
10. Choi, J., Fauce, S.R., Effros, R.B. "Reduced telomerase activity in human T lymphocytes exposed to cortisol." *Brain, Behavior, and Immunity* 22.4 (2008):600–5.
11. Kroenke, C.H., Epel, E., Adler, N., Bush, N.R., et al. "Autonomic and adrenocortical reactivity and buccal cell telomere length in kindergarten children." *Psychosomatic Medicine*

73.7 (2011):533–40.

12. Konturek, P.C., Brzozowski, T., Konturek S.J. "Stress and the gut: pathophysiology, clinical consequences, diagnostic approach and treatment options." *Journal of Physiological Pharmacology* 62.6 (2011):591–9.

13. Cohen, S., et al. "Chronic stress, glucocorticoid receptor resistance, inflammation, and disease risk." *Proceedings of the National Academy of Sciences of the United States of America* 109.16 (2012):5995–99. PMC. Web. 18 Aug. 2017.

14. Sulkowski, M.L., Dempsey, J., Dempsey, A.G. "Effects of stress and coping on binge eating in female college students." *Eating Behaviors* 12.3 (2011):188–91.

15. Nevanperä, N.J., et al. "Occupational burnout, eating behavior, and weight among working women." *The American Journal of Clinical Nutrition* 95.4 (2012):934–43.

16. Moore, C.J., Cunningham, S.A. "Social position, psychological stress, and obesity: a systematic review." *Journal of the Academy of Nutrition and Dietetics* 112.4 (2012):518–26.

17. Kivimäki, M., et al. "Work stress, weight gain and weight loss: evidence for bidirectional effects of job strain on body mass index in the Whitehall II study." *International Journal of Obesity* 30.6 (2006):982–7.

18. Ansell, E.B. et al. "Cumulative adversity and smaller gray matter volume in medial prefrontal, anterior cingulate, and insula regions." *Biological Psychiatry* 72.1 (2012):57–64. PMC. Web. 18 Aug. 2017.

19. Chetty, S., et al. "Stress and glucocorticoids promote oligodendrogenesis in the adult hippocampus." *Molecular Psychiatry* 19.12 (2014):1275–83.

20. Marmot, M.G., et al. "Employment grade and coronary heart disease in British civil servants." *Journal of Epidemiology & Community Health* 32.4 (1978):244–49.

21. Marmot, M.G., et al. "Health inequalities among British civil servants: the Whitehall II study." *The Lancet* 337.8754 (1991):1387–93.

21a. Anderson, Norman B., et al. "Stress in America: paying with our health." American Psychological Association (2015).

22. Hintsa, T., et al. "Higher effort-reward imbalance and lower job control predict exit from the labour market at the age of 61 years or younger: evidence from the English Longitudinal Study of Ageing." *Journal of Epidemiology and Community Health* 69.6 (2015):543–9.

23. Bonde, J.P.E. "Psychosocial factors at work and risk of depression: a systematic review of the epidemiological evidence." *Occupational and Environmental Medicine* 65.7 (2008):438–45.

24. Stansfeld, S.A., Head, J., Marmot, M.G. *Work-related factors and ill health: the Whitehall II study.* Sudbury: HSE Books, 2000.

25. De Vogli, R., et al. "Unfairness and health: evidence from the Whitehall II Study." *Journal of Epidemiology & Community Health* 61.6 (2007):513–18.

26. Kivimäki, M., et al. "Organisational justice and health of employees: prospective cohort study." *Occupational and Environmental Medicine* 60.1 (2003):27–34.

27. Van Vegchel, N., et al. "Reviewing the effort-reward imbalance model: drawing up the balance of 45 empirical studies." *Social Science & Medicine* 60.5 (2005):1117–31.

28. Kuper, H., et al. "When reciprocity fails: effort-reward imbalance in relation to coronary heart disease and health functioning within the Whitehall II study." *Occupational and Environmental Medicine* 59.11 (2002):777–84.

29. Siegrist, J., et al. "The measurement of effort-reward imbalance at work: European comparisons." *Social Science & Medicine* 58.8 (2004):1483–99.

30. World Health Organization. "Depression and other common mental disorders: global health estimates." (2017).

31. Vos, T., et al. "Global, regional, and national incidence, prevalence, and years lived with disability for 310 diseases and injuries, 1990–2015: a systematic analysis for the Global Burden of Disease Study 2015." *The Lancet* 388.10053 (2016):1545–1602.

32. Garatachea, N., et al. "Elite athletes live longer than the general population: a meta-analysis." *Mayo Clinic Proceedings* 89.9 (2014):1195–200.

33. Kettunen, J.A., et al. "All-cause and disease-specific mortality among male, former elite athletes: an average 50-year follow-up." *British Journal of Sports Medicine* 49.13 (2015):893–7.

34. Zwiers, R., et al. "Mortality in former Olympic athletes: retrospective cohort analysis." *BMJ* 345 (2012):e7456.

35. Keller, A., et al. "Does the perception that stress affects health matter? The association with health and mortality." *Health Psychology* 31.5 (2012):677–84.

36. Jamieson, J.P., Nock, M.K., Mendes, W.B. "Mind over matter: reappraising arousal improves cardiovascular and cognitive responses to stress." *Journal of Experimental Psychology: General* 141.3 (2012):417–22.

37. Jamieson, J.P., Nock, M.K., Mendes, W.B. "Changing the conceptualization of stress in social anxiety disorder: Affective and physiological consequences." *Clinical Psychological Science* 1.4 (2013):363–74.

38. Jamieson, J.P., et al. "Turning the knots in your stomach into bows: Reappraising arousal improves performance on the GRE." *Journal of Experimental Social Psychology* 46.1 (2010):208–12.

39. Olff, M., et al. "The role of oxytocin in social bonding, stress regulation and mental health: an update on the moderating effects of context and interindividual differences." *Psychoneuroendocrinology* 38.9 (2013):1883–94.

40. LeDoux, J.E. "The amygdala: contributions to fear and stress." *Seminars in Neuroscience* 6.4 (1994):231–37.

41. Uvnas-Moberg, K., Petersson, M. "Oxytocin, a mediator of anti-stress, well-being, social interaction, growth and healing." *Zeitschrift für Psychosomatische Medizin und Psychotherapie* 51.1 (2005):57–80.

42. Taylor, S.E. "Tend and befriend: biobehavioral bases of affiliation under stress." *Current Directions in Psychological Science* 15.6 (2006):273–7.

43. Poulin, M.J., et al. "Giving to others and the association between stress and mortality." *American Journal of Public Health* 103.9 (2013):1649–55.

44. Poulin, M.J., Holman, E.A. "Helping hands, healthy body? Oxytocin receptor gene and prosocial behavior interact to buffer the association between stress and physical health." *Hormones and Behavior* 63.3 (2013):510–7.

45. Stellar, J.E., et al. "Affective and physiological responses to the suffering of others: compassion and vagal activity." *Journal of Personality and Social Psychology* 108.4 (2015):572–85.

46. Floyd, K., et al. "Human affection exchange: XIV. Relational affection predicts resting heart rate and free cortisol secretion during acute stress." *Behavioral Medicine* 32.4 (2007):151–56.

47. Floyd, K., et al. "Human affection exchange: XIII. Affectionate communication accelerates neuroendocrine stress recovery." *Health Communication* 22.2 (2007):123–32.

48. Taylor, S.E., Klein, L.C., Lewis, B.P., Gruenewald, T.L., Gurung, R.A., Updegraff, J.A. "Biobehavioral responses to stress in females: tend-and-befriend, not fight-or-flight." *Psychological Review.* 107.3 (2000):411–29.

49. Preston, S.D. "The origins of altruism in offspring care." *Psychological Bulletin* 139.6 (2013):1305–41.

50. Diamond, L.M., Fagundes, C.P., Butterworth, M.R. "Attachment style, vagal tone, and empathy during mother-adolescent interactions." *Journal of Research on Adolescence* 22.1 (2012):165–84.

51. Bonaz, B., Sinniger, V., Pellissier, S. "Anti–inflammatory properties of the vagus nerve: potential therapeutic implications of vagus nerve stimulation." *The Journal of Physiology* 594.20 (2016):5781–90.

52. Olson, K.L., et al. "The hypothalamic-pituitary-adrenal axis: the actions of the central nervous system and potential biomarkers." *Anti-Aging Therapeutics* 13 (2011):91–100

53. Tracey, K.J. "The inflammatory reflex." *Nature* 420.6917 (2002):853–9.

54. Koopman, F.A., et al. "Vagus nerve stimulation inhibits cytokine production and attenuates disease severity in rheumatoid arthritis." *Proceedings of the National Academy of Sciences* 113.29 (2016):8284–89.

55. Sinniger, V., et al. "Electrical vagus nerve stimulation as an innovative treatment in inflammatory bowel diseases." *Journal of Crohn's and Colitis.* Vol. 10. Oxford University Press, 2016.

56. Vonck, K., et al. "Vagus nerve stimulation ... 25 years later! What do we know about the effects on cognition?" *Neuroscience & Biobehavioral Reviews* 45 (2014):63–71.

57. Pellissier, S., et al. "Relationship between vagal tone, cortisol, TNF-alpha, epinephrine and negative affects in Crohn's disease and irritable bowel syndrome." *PLOS ONE* 9.9 (2014):e105328.

58. Green, L.A., Weaver, D.F. "Vagal stimulation by manual carotid sinus massage to acutely suppress seizures." *Journal of Clinical Neuroscience* 21.1 (2014):179–80.

59. Diego, M.A., Field, T., Hernandez-Reif, M. "Vagal activity, gastric motility and weight gain in massaged preterm neonates." *Journal of Pediatrics* 147.1 (2005):50–5.

60. Field, T., et al. "Cortisol decreases and serotonin and dopamine increase following massage therapy." *International Journal of Neuroscience* 115.10 (2005):1397–1413.

61. Lehrer, P.M., Gevirtz, R. "Heart rate variability biofeedback: how and why does it work?" *Frontiers in Psychology* 5 (2014).

62. Lin, G., Xiang, Q., Fu, X., Wang, S., Wang, S., Chen, S., et al. "Heart rate variability biofeedback decreases blood pressure in prehypertensive subjects by improving autonomic function and baroreflex." *Journal of Alternative and Complementary Medicine* 18 (2012):143–52. doi: 10.1089/acm.2010.0607.

63. Grundy, D. "Neuroanatomy of visceral nociception: vagal and splanchnic afferent." *Gut* 51.Suppl 1 (2002):i2–i5.

64. Mason, H., et al. "Cardiovascular and respiratory effect of yogic slow breathing in the yoga beginner: what is the best approach?" *Journal of Evidence-Based Complementary and Alternative Medicine* (2013).

65. Lin, I.M., Tai, L.Y., Fan, S.Y. "Breathing at a rate of 5.5 breaths per minute with equal inhalation-to-exhalation ratio increases heart rate variability." *International Journal of Psychophysiology* 91.3 (2014):206–11.

66. Lindholm, P., Lundgren, Claes E.G. "The physiology and pathophysiology of human breath-hold diving." *Journal of Applied Physiology* 106.1 (2009):284–92.
67. Kinoshita, T., et al. "Cold-water face immersion per se elicits cardiac parasympathetic activity." *Circulation Journal*: official journal of the Japanese Circulation Society 70.6 (2006):773–6.
68. Chase, N.L., Sui, X., Blair, S.N. "Swimming and all-cause mortality risk compared with running, walking, and sedentary habits in men." *International Journal of Aquatic Research and Education* 2.3 (2008):213–23.
69. Sant'Ana, J.E., et al. "Effect of the duration of daily aerobic physical training on cardiac autonomic adaptations." *Autonomic Neuroscience* 159.1 (2011):32–7.
70. Kinoshita, T., et al. "Cold-water face immersion per se elicits cardiac parasympathetic activity." *Circulation Journal* 70.6 (2006):773–6.
71. Khurana, R.K., Wu, R. "The Cold Face Test: a non-baroreflex mediated test of cardiac vagal function." *Clinical Autonomic Research* 16.3 (2006): 202–7.
72. Lemaitre, F., Chowdhury, T., Schaller, B. "The trigeminocardiac reflex – a comparison with the diving reflex in humans." *Archives of Medical Science*: AMS 11.2 (2015):419–26. PMC. Web. 13 Sept. 2017.
73. Schaller, B., et al. "Trigeminocardiac reflex during surgery in the cerebellopontine angle." *Journal of Neurosurgery* 90.2 (1999):215–20.
74. La Marca, R., et al. "Association between Cold Face Test-induced vagal inhibition and cortisol response to acute stress." *Psychophysiology* 48.3 (2011):420–29.
75. Tyagi, A., Cohen, M. "Yoga and heart rate variability: a comprehensive review of the literature." *International Journal of Yoga* 9.2 (2016):97–113. PMC. Web. 17 Sept. 2017.
76. Sharma, M. "Yoga as an alternative and complementary approach for stress management: a systematic review." *Journal of Evidence-Based Complementary and Alternative Medicine* 19.1 (2014):59–67.
77. Li, A.W., Goldsmith, C.A. "The effects of yoga on anxiety and stress." *Alternative Medicine Review* 17.1 (2012):21–35.
78. Butzer, B., et al. "Effects of a classroom-based yoga intervention on cortisol and behavior in second- and third-grade students: a pilot study." *Journal of Evidence-Based Complementary and Alternative Medicine* 20.1 (2015):41–9. PMC. Web. 17 Sept. 2017.
79. Thirthalli, J. et al. "Cortisol and antidepressant effects of yoga." *Indian Journal of Psychiatry* 55.Suppl 3 (2013):S405–8. PMC. Web. 18 Sept. 2017.
80. Pandey, P.T., Singh, V., Haider, J. "Effect of yoga on salivary cortisol in medical students." *International Journal of Research in Medical Sciences* 4.11 (2016):4995–8.
81. Jacobs, T.L., et al. "Self-reported mindfulness and cortisol during a Shamatha meditation retreat." *Health Psychology* 32.10 (2013):1104–9.
82. University of Oregon. "Body-mind Meditation Boosts Performance, Reduces Stress." *ScienceDaily*, 9 October 2007.
83. Hoge, E.A., et al. "The effect of mindfulness meditation training on biological acute stress responses in generalized anxiety disorder." *Psychiatry Research* 262 (2017):328–32.
84. Fox, K.C.R., et al. "Is meditation associated with altered brain structure? A systematic review and meta-analysis of morphometric neuroimaging in meditation practitioners." *Neuroscience & Biobehavioral Reviews* 43 (2014):48–73.
85. Hölzel, B.K., et al. "Mindfulness practice leads to increases in regional brain gray matter

density." *Psychiatry Research: Neuroimaging* 191.1 (2011):36–43.

86. Luders, Eileen, et al. "Forever young(er): potential age-defying effects of long-term meditation on gray matter atrophy." *Deutsche Zeitschrift für Akupunktur* 58.4 (2015):30–1.

87. Peters, R. "Ageing and the brain." *Postgraduate Medical Journal* 82.964 (2006):84–8. PMC. Web. 8 Apr. 2018.

88. Pagnoni, G., Cekic, M. "Age effects on gray matter volume and attentional performance in Zen meditation." *Neurobiological Aging* 28, (2007):1623–27. doi: 10.1016/j.neurobiolaging.2007.06.008.

89. Tang, Yi-Yuan, et al. "Brief mental training reorganizes large-scale brain networks." *Frontiers in Systems Neuroscience* 11 (2017).

90. Creswell, J.D., Lindsay, E.K. "How does mindfulness training affect health? A mindfulness stress buffering account. *Current Directions in Psychological Science* 23.6 (2014):401–7.

91. Arnsten, A.F.T. "Stress signalling pathways that impair prefrontal cortex structure and function." *Nature Reviews Neuroscience* 10 (2009):410–22.

92. Slavich, G.M., Irwin, M.R. "From stress to inflammation and major depressive disorder: A social signal transduction theory of depression." *Psychological Bulletin* 140.3 (2014):774–815.

93. Buric, I., et al. "What is the molecular signature of mind-body interventions? A systematic review of gene expression changes induced by meditation and related practices." *Frontiers in Immunology* 8 (2017).

94. Black, D.S., et al. "Yogic meditation reverses NF-κB and IRF-related transcriptome dynamics in leukocytes of family dementia caregivers in a randomized controlled trial." *Psychoneuroendocrinology* 38.3 (2013):348–55.

95. Fox, K.C.R., et al. "Functional neuroanatomy of meditation: a review and meta-analysis of 78 functional neuroimaging investigations." *Neuroscience & Biobehavioral Reviews* 65 (2016):208–28.

96. Tang, Yi-Yuan. "Mechanism of integrative body-mind training." *Neuroscience Bulletin* 27.6 (2011):383–8.

97. Lutz, A., et al. "Attention regulation and monitoring in meditation." *Trends in Cognitive Sciences* 12.4 (2008):163–9.

98. Hyman, J.M., Holroyd, C.B., Seamans, J.K. "A novel neural prediction error found in anterior cingulate cortex ensembles." *Neuron* 95.2 (2017):447–56.

99. Leiberg, S., Klimecki, O., Singer, T. "Short-term compassion training increases prosocial behavior in a newly developed prosocial game." *PLOS ONE* 6.3 (2011):e17798.

100. Terry, P.C., et al. "Effects of synchronous music on treadmill running among elite triathletes." *Journal of Science and Medicine in Sport* 15.1 (2012):52–7.

101. Roerdink, M. "Anchoring: moving from theory to therapy." (2009). Research report.

102. Chanda, M.L., Levitin, D.J. "The neurochemistry of music." *Trends in Cognitive Sciences* 17.4 (2013):179–93.

103. Menon, V., Levitin, D.J. "The rewards of music listening: response and physiological connectivity of the mesolimbic system." *NeuroImage* 28.1 (2005):175–84.

104. Latha, R., et al. "Effect of music on heart rate variability and stress in medical students." *International Journal of Clinical and Experimental Physiology* 1.2 (2014):131–4.

105. Nilsson, U. "Soothing music can increase oxytocin levels during bed rest after open–heart surgery: a randomised control trial." *Journal of Clinical Nursing* 18.15 (2009):2153–61.

106. Fancourt, D., Ockelford, A., Belai, A. "The psychoneuroimmunological effects of music:

a systematic review and a new model." *Brain, Behavior, and Immunity* 36 (2014):15–26.

107. Gerra, G., et al. "Neuroendocrine responses of healthy volunteers to techno-music: relationships with personality traits and emotional state." *International Journal of Psychophysiology* 28.1 (1998):99–111.

108. Thoma, M.V., et al. "The effect of music on the human stress response." Ed. Robert L. Newton. *PLOS ONE* 8.8 (2013):e70156. PMC. Web. 25 Mar. 2018.

109. McEwen, B.S., Karatsoreos, I.N. "Sleep deprivation and circadian disruption: stress, allostasis, and allostatic load." *Sleep Medicine Clinics* 10.1 (2015):1–10.

110. Wang, Q., et al. "The effects of music intervention on sleep quality in community-dwelling elderly." *The Journal of Alternative and Complementary Medicine* 22.7 (2016):576–84.

111. Feng, F., et al. "Can music improve sleep quality in adults with primary insomnia? A systematic review and network meta-analysis." *International Journal of Nursing Studies* 77 (2018):189–96.

112. Verrusio, W., et al. "The Mozart effect: a quantitative EEG study." *Consciousness and Cognition* 35 (2015):150–5.

113. Jacobs, G.D., Friedman, R. "EEG spectral analysis of relaxation techniques." *Applied Psychophysiology and Biofeedback* 29.4 (2004).

114. Tsujita, S., Morimoto, K. "Secretory IgA in saliva can be a useful stress marker." *Environmental Health and Preventive Medicine* 4.1 (1999):1–8. PMC. Web. 27 Apr. 2018.

115. Fujimaru, C., et al. "Self–perceived work–related stress and its relation to salivary IgA, cortisol and 3–methoxy–4–hydroxyphenyl glycol levels among neonatal intensive care nurses." *Stress and Health* 28.2 (2012):171–4.

116. Yang, Y., et al. "Self-perceived work related stress and the relation with salivary IgA and lysozyme among emergency department nurses." *Occupational and Environmental Medicine* 59.12 (2002):836–41.

117. Kejr, A., et al. "Receptive music therapy and salivary histamine secretion." *Inflammation Research* 59.2 (2010):217–18.

118. Gabay, C. "Interleukin-6 and chronic inflammation." *Arthritis Research & Therapy* 8.Suppl 2 (2006):S3. PMC. Web. 29 Apr. 2018.

119. Okada, K., et al. "Effects of music therapy on autonomic nervous system activity, incidence of heart failure events, and plasma cytokine and catecholamine levels in elderly patients with cerebrovascular disease and dementia." *International Heart Journal* 50.1 (2009):95–110.

120. Conrad, C., et al. "Overture for growth hormone: requiem for interleukin-6?" *Critical Care Medicine* 35.12 (2007):2709–13.

121. Bouchard-Mercier, A., et al. "Associations between dietary patterns and gene expression profiles of healthy men and women: a cross-sectional study." *Nutrition Journal* 12 (2013):24. PMC. Web. 1 Jan. 2018.

122. Van Dijk, S.J., et al. "A saturated fatty acid-rich diet induces an obesity-linked proinflammatory gene expression profile in adipose tissue of subjects at risk of metabolic syndrome." *The American Journal of Clinical Nutrition* 90.6 (2009):1656–64.

123. Gjevestad, G.O., Holven, K.B., Ulven, S.M. "Effects of exercise on gene expression of inflammatory markers in human peripheral blood cells: a systematic review." *Current Cardiovascular Risk Reports* 9.7 (2015):34. PMC. Web. 1 Jan. 2018.

124. Ratey, J.J., Hagerman, E., Ratey, J. *Spark: how exercise will improve the performance of your*

brain. Hachette UK, 2010.

125. Berchtold, N. C., et al. "Exercise primes a molecular memory for brain-derived neurotrophic factor protein induction in the rat hippocampus." *Neuroscience* 133.3 (2005):853–61.

126. Marquez, C.M.S., et al. "High-intensity interval training evokes larger serum BDNF levels compared with intense continuous exercise." *Journal of Applied Physiology* 119.12 (2015):1363–73.

127. Goekint, M., et al. "Influence of citalopram and environmental temperature on exercise-induced changes in BDNF." *Neuroscience Letters* 494.2 (2011):150–4.

128. Church, D.D., et al. "Comparison of high-intensity vs. high-volume resistance training on the BDNF response to exercise." *Journal of Applied Physiology* 121.1 (2016):123–8.

129. Correia, P.R., Pansani, A., Machado, F., Andrade, M., Silva da, A.C., Scorza, F.A., Cavalheiro, E.A., Arida, R.M. "Acute strength exercise and the involvement of small or large muscle mass on plasma brain-derived neurotrophic factor levels." *Clinics* 65 (2010):1123–6.

130. Seifert, T., et al. "Endurance training enhances BDNF release from the human brain." *American Journal of Physiology – Regulatory, Integrative and Comparative Physiology* 298.2 (2009):R372–7.

131. Schmolesky, M.T., Webb, D.L., Hansen, R.A. "The effects of aerobic exercise intensity and duration on levels of brain-derived neurotrophic factor in healthy men." *Journal of Sports Science and Medicine* 12.3 (2013):502–11.

132. Goldenberg, N., Barkan, A. "Factors regulating growth hormone secretion in humans." *Endocrinology Metabolism Clinics of North America* 36.1 (2007):37–55.

133. Consitt, L.A., Bloomer, R.J., Wideman, L. "The effect of exercise type on immunofunctional and traditional growth hormone." *European Journal of Applied Physiology* 100.3 (2007):321–30.

134. Thomas, G.A., et al. "Obesity, growth hormone and exercise." *Sports Medicine* 43.9 (2013):839–49.

135. Felsing, N.E., Brasel, J.A., Cooper, D.M. "Effect of low and high intensity exercise on circulating growth hormone in men." *Journal of Clinical Endocrinology & Metabolism* 75.1 (1992):157–62.

136. Nindl, B.C., et al. "Twenty-hour growth hormone secretory profiles after aerobic and resistance exercise." *Medicine and Science in Sports and Exercise* 46.10 (2014):1917–27.

137. Seifert, T., et al. "Endurance training enhances BDNF release from the human brain." *American Journal of Physiology – Regulatory, Integrative and Comparative Physiology* 298.2 (2009):R372–7.

138. Gillen, J.B., et al. "Three minutes of all-out intermittent exercise per week increases skeletal muscle oxidative capacity and improves cardiometabolic health." *PLOS ONE* 9.11 (2014):e111489.

139. Gillen, J.B., et al. "Twelve weeks of sprint interval training improves indices of cardiometabolic health similar to traditional endurance training despite a five-fold lower exercise volume and time commitment." *PLOS ONE* 11.4 (2016):e0154075.

140. Fell, G.L., et al. "Skin β-endorphin mediates addiction to UV light." *Cell* 157.7 (2014):1527–34.

141. Dopico, X.C., et al. "Widespread seasonal gene expression reveals annual differences in

human immunity and physiology." *Nature Communications* 6, Article 7000 (2015).

142. Liu, D., et al. "UVA irradiation of human skin vasodilates arterial vasculature and lowers blood pressure independently of nitric oxide synthase." *Journal of Investigative Dermatology* 134.7 (2014):1839–46.

143. Van der Rhee, H., et al. "Sunlight: For better or for worse? A review of positive and negative effects of sun exposure." *Cancer Research Frontiers* 2 (2016):156–83.

144. Lindqvist, P.G., et al. "Avoidance of sun exposure as a risk factor for major causes of death: a competing risk analysis of the Melanoma in Southern Sweden cohort." *Journal of Internal Medicine* 280.4 (2016):375–87.

145. Phan, T.X., et al. "Intrinsic photosensitivity enhances motility of T lymphocytes." *Scientific Reports* 6, Article 39479 (2016).

146. Wang, Ya., et al. "UV light selectively inhibits spinal cord inflammation and demyelination in experimental autoimmune encephalomyelitis." *Archives of Biochemistry and Biophysics* 567 (2015):75–82.

147. Molendijk, M.L., et al. "Serum BDNF concentrations show strong seasonal variation and correlations with the amount of ambient sunlight." *PLOS ONE* 7.11 (2012):e48046.

148. Patrick, R.P., Ames, B.N. "Vitamin D hormone regulates serotonin synthesis. Part 1: relevance for autism." *The FASEB Journal* 28.6 (2014):2398–2413.

149. Hoel, D.G., et al. "The risks and benefits of sun exposure 2016." *Dermato-Endocrinology* 8.1 (2016):e1248325.

150. Katare, R.G., et al. "Chronic intermittent fasting improves the survival following large myocardial ischemia by activation of BDNF/VEGF/PI3K signaling pathway." *Journal of Molecular and Cellular Cardiology* 46.3 (2009):405–12.

151. Walsh, J.J., et al. "Fasting and exercise differentially regulate BDNF mRNA expression in human skeletal muscle." *Applied Physiology, Nutrition, and Metabolism* 40.1 (2014):96–8.

152. Hartman, M.L., et al. "Augmented growth hormone (GH) secretory burst frequency and amplitude mediate enhanced GH secretion during a two-day fast in normal men." *Journal of Clinical Endocrinology & Metabolism* 74.4 (1992):757–65.

153. Intermountain Medical Center. "Routine periodic fasting is good for your health, and your heart, study suggests." *ScienceDaily*, 20 May 2011. www.sciencedaily.com/releases/2011/04/110403090259.htm

154. Horne, B.D., et al. "Randomized cross-over trial of short-term water-only fasting: metabolic and cardiovascular consequences." *Nutrition, Metabolism and Cardiovascular Diseases* 23.11 (2013):1050–7.

155. Longo, V.D., Mattson, M.P. "Fasting: molecular mechanisms and clinical applications." *Cell Metabolism* 19.2 (2014):181–92.

156. Stranahan, A.M., et al. "Voluntary exercise and caloric restriction enhance hippocampal dendritic spine density and BDNF levels in diabetic mice." *Hippocampus* 19.10 (2009):951–61.

157. Kishi, T., et al. "Calorie restriction improves cognitive decline via up-regulation of brain-derived neurotrophic factor." *International Heart Journal* 56.1 (2015):110–5.

158. Holloszy, J.O., et al. "Effect of voluntary exercise on longevity of rats." *Journal of Applied Physiology* 59.3 (1985):826–31.

159. Willcox, B.J., D.C. Willcox. "Caloric restriction, caloric restriction mimetics, and healthy aging in Okinawa: controversies and clinical implications." *Current Opinion in Clinical*

Nutrition and Metabolic Care 17.1 (2014):51–8.

160. Breese, C.R., Ingram, R.L., Sonntag, W.E. "Influence of age and long-term dietary restriction on plasma insulin-like growth factor-1 (IGF-1), IGF-1 gene expression, and IGF-1 binding proteins." *Journal of Gerontology* 46.5 (1991):B180–7.

161. Sabatino, F., et al. "Assessment of the role of the glucocorticoid system in aging processes and in the action of food restriction." *Journal of Gerontology* 46.5 (1991):B171–9.

162. Weiss, E.P., et al. "Improvements in glucose tolerance and insulin action induced by increasing energy expenditure or decreasing energy intake: a randomized controlled trial." *The American Journal of Clinical Nutrition* 84.5 (2006):1033–42.

163. Fontana, L., et al. "Long–term effects of calorie or protein restriction on serum IGF–1 and IGFBP–3 concentration in humans." *Aging Cell* 7.5 (2008):681–7.

164. Tam, C.S., et al. "No effect of caloric restriction on salivary cortisol levels in overweight men and women." *Metabolism* 63.2 (2014):194–8.

165. Abedelmalek, S., et al. "Caloric restriction effect on proinflammatory cytokines, growth hormone, and steroid hormone concentrations during exercise in Judokas." *Oxidative Medicine and Cellular Longevity* 2015 (2015).

166. Kulkarni, S.K., Dhir, A. "An overview of curcumin in neurological disorders." *Indian Journal of Pharmaceutical Sciences* 72.2 (2010):149–54.

167. Zhang, L., et al. "Effects of curcumin on chronic, unpredictable, mild, stress-induced depressive-like behaviour and structural plasticity in the lateral amygdala of rats." *International Journal of Neuropsychopharmacology* 17.5 (2014):793–806.

168. Huang, Z., et al. "Curcumin reverses corticosterone-induced depressive-like behavior and decrease in brain BDNF levels in rats." *Neuroscience Letters* 493.3 (2011):145–8.

169. Li, Yu-Cheng, et al. "Antidepressant-like effects of curcumin on serotonergic receptor-coupled AC-cAMP pathway in chronic unpredictable mild stress of rats." *Progress in Neuro-Psychopharmacology and Biological Psychiatry* 33.3 (2009):435–49.

170. Lopresti, A.L., Hood, S.D., Drummond, P.D. "Multiple antidepressant potential modes of action of curcumin: a review of its anti-inflammatory, monoaminergic, antioxidant, immune-modulating and neuroprotective effects." *Journal of Psychopharmacology* (2012):0269881112458732.

171. Lao, C.D., et al. "Dose escalation of a curcuminoid formulation." *BMC Complementary and Alternative Medicine.* (2006).

172. Sasaki, H., et al. "Innovative preparation of curcumin for improved oral bioavailability." *Biological and Pharmaceutical Bulletin* 34.5 (2011):660–5.

173. Cuomo, J., et al. "Comparative absorption of a standardized curcuminoid mixture and its lecithin formulation." *Journal of Natural Products* 74.4 (2011):664–9.

174. Lechtenberg, M., Quandt, B., Nahrstedt, A. "Quantitative determination of curcuminoids in Curcuma rhizomes and rapid differentiation of Curcuma domestica Val. and Curcuma xanthorrhiza Roxb. by capillary electrophoresis." *Phytochemical Analysis*: PCA 15.3 (2004):152–8.

175. Nakayama, H., et al. "A single consumption of curry improved post-prandial endothelial function in healthy male subjects: a randomized, controlled crossover trial." *Nutrition Journal.* (2014)

176. Srivastava, K.C., Bordia, A., Verma, S.K. "Curcumin, a major component of food spice turmeric (Curcuma longa) inhibits aggregation and alters eicosanoid metabolism

in human blood platelets." *Prostaglandins, Leukotrienes and Essential Fatty Acids* 52.4 (1995):223–7.

177. Qiu, P., et al. "Overdose intake of curcumin initiates the unbalanced state of bodies." *Journal of Agricultural and Food Chemistry* 64.13 (2016):2765–71.

178. Gambini J., Inglés M., Olaso G., et al. "Properties of resveratrol: in vitro and in vivo studies about metabolism, bioavailability, and biological effects in animal models and humans." *Oxidative Medicine and Cellular Longevity* 2015:837042 (2015). doi:10.1155/2015/837042.

179. Wang, X., et al. "Resveratrol reverses chronic restraint stress-induced depression-like behaviour: involvement of BDNF level, ERK phosphorylation and expression of Bcl-2 and Bax in rats." *Brain Research Bulletin* 125 (2016):134–43.

180. Hurley, L.L., et al. "Antidepressant effects of resveratrol in an animal model of depression." *Behavioural Brain Research* 268 (2014):1–7.

181. Ge, Jin-Fang, et al. "Antidepressant-like effect of resveratrol: involvement of antioxidant effect and peripheral regulation on HPA axis." *Pharmacology Biochemistry and Behavior* 114 (2013):64–9.

182. Albani, D., et al. "Neuroprotective properties of resveratrol in different neurodegenerative disorders." *Biofactors* 36.5 (2010):370–6.

183. Xu, Y., et al. "Antidepressant-like effect of trans-resveratrol: involvement of serotonin and noradrenaline system." *European Neuropsychopharmacology* 20.6 (2010):405–13.

184. Patel, K.R., et al. "Clinical trials of resveratrol." *Annals of the New York Academy of Sciences*, 1215 (2011):161–9.

185. Chow, H.H. Sherry, et al. "Resveratrol modulates drug-and carcinogen-metabolizing enzymes in a healthy volunteer study." *Cancer Prevention Research* 3.9 (2010):1168–75.

186. Almeida, L., et al. "Pharmacokinetic and safety profile of trans–resveratrol in a rising multiple–dose study in healthy volunteers." *Molecular Nutrition & Food Research* 53.S1 (2009).

187. La Porte, C., et al. "Steady-State pharmacokinetics and tolerability of trans-resveratrol 2000 mg twice daily with food, quercetin and alcohol (ethanol) in healthy human subjects." *Clinical Pharmacokinetics.* (2010).

188. Simopoulos, A.P. "The importance of the omega-6/omega-3 fatty acid ratio in cardiovascular disease and other chronic diseases." *Experimental Biology and Medicine* 233.6 (2008):674–88.

189. Sanders, T.A. "Polyunsaturated fatty acids in the food chain in Europe." *The American Journal of Clinical Nutrition* 71.Suppl 1 (2000):176–8.

190. Sugano, M., Hirahara, F. "Polyunsaturated fatty acids in the food chain in Japan." *The American Journal of Clinical Nutrition* 71.Suppl 1 (2000):189–96.

191. Danaei, G., et al. "The preventable causes of death in the United States: comparative risk assessment of dietary, lifestyle, and metabolic risk factors." *PLOS ONE* 6.4 (2009):e1000058.

192. Delarue, J.O.C.P., et al. "Fish oil prevents the adrenal activation elicited by mental stress in healthy men." *Diabetes & Metabolism* 29.3 (2003):289–95.

193. Pusceddu, M.M., et al. "The Omega-3 polyunsaturated fatty acid docosahexaenoic acid (DHA) reverses corticosterone-induced changes in cortical neurons." *International Journal of Neuropsychopharmacology* 19.6 (2016):pyv130.

194. Witte, V.A., et al. "Long-chain omega-3 fatty acids improve brain function and structure

in older adults." *Cerebral Cortex* (2013):bht163.

195. Van de Rest, O., et al. "Effect of fish oil on cognitive performance in older subjects: a randomized, controlled trial." *Neurology* 71.6 (2008):430–8.

196. Yan, Y., et al. "Omega-3 fatty acids prevent inflammation and metabolic disorder through inhibition of NLRP3 inflammasome activation." *Immunity* 38.6 (2013):1154–63.

197. Patrick, R.P., Ames, B.N. "Vitamin D and the omega-3 fatty acids control serotonin synthesis and action, part 2: relevance for ADHD, bipolar, schizophrenia, and impulsive behavior." *The FASEB Journal* 29.6 (2015):2207–22.

198. http://www.who.int/en/news-room/fact-sheets/detail/mercury-and-health

199. https://www.epa.gov/mercury/health-effects-exposures-mercury

200. Kris-Etherton, P.M., Harris, W.S., Appel, L.J. "Fish consumption, fish oil, omega-3 fatty acids, and cardiovascular disease." *Circulation* 106.21 (2002):2747–57.

201. Hightower, J.M., Moore, D. "Mercury levels in high-end consumers of fish." *Environmental Health Perspectives* 111.4 (2003):604–8.

202. Sidhu, K.S. "Health benefits and potential risks related to consumption of fish or fish oil." *Regulatory Toxicology and Pharmacology* 38.3 (2003):336–44.

203. https://www.csir.co.za/csir-research-mercury-fish-informs-consumer-choices

204. *Nutrition Business Journal.* NBJ's Supplement Business Report 2015. Penton Media, Inc., 2015.

205. Schlebusch, L., et al. "A double-blind, placebo-controlled, double-centre study of the effects of an oral multivitamin-mineral combination on stress." *South African Medical Journal* 90.12 (2000):1216–23.

206. Carroll, D., Ring, C., Suter, M., Willemsen, G. "The effects of an oral multivitamin combination with calcium, magnesium, and zinc on psychological well-being in healthy young male volunteers: a double-blind placebo-controlled trial." *Psychopharmacology* 150.2 (2000):220–5. 10.1007/s002130000406.

207. Long, S., Benton, D. "Effects of vitamin and mineral supplementation on stress, mild psychiatric symptoms, and mood in nonclinical samples: a meta-analysis." *Psychosomatic Medicine* 75.2 (2013):144–53.

208. Stoney, C.M. "Plasma homocysteine levels increase in women during psychological stress." *Life Sciences* 64.25 (1999):2359–65.

209. Ford, A.H., Flicker, L., Urvashnee, S., Hirani, V., Almeida, O.P. "Homocysteine, depression and cognitive function in older adults." *Journal of Affective Disorders* 151.2 (2013):646–51. 10.1016/j.jad.2013.07.012.

210. Lodhi, R., Aashish, P. "Interrelationship of Vitamin B12, Androgens and Cortisol in Chronic Stress and Associated Vascular Dysfunction." *Journal of Pharmaceutical Science and Bioscientific Research* 4.5 (2014):293–334.

211. Tangney, C.C., Aggarwal, N.T., Li, H., Wilson, R.S., De Carli, C., Evans, D.A., Morris, M.C. "Vitamin B12, cognition, and brain MRI measures. A cross-sectional examination." *Neurology* 77.13 (2011):1276–82. 10.1212/WNL.0b013e3182315a33.

212. Smith, D.A., et al. "Homocysteine-lowering by B vitamins slows the rate of accelerated brain atrophy in mild cognitive impairment: a randomized controlled trial." *PLOS ONE* 5.9 (2010):e12244.

213. Stough, C., et al. "The effect of 90 day administration of a high dose vitamin B–complex on work stress." *Human Psychopharmacology: Clinical and Experimental* 26.7 (2011):470–6.

214. Sachs, B.D., Ni, J.R., Caron, M.G. "Brain 5-HT deficiency increases stress vulnerability and impairs antidepressant responses following psychosocial stress." *Proceedings of the National Academy of Sciences* 112.8 (2015):2557–62.

215. Davis, M.T., et al. "Neurobiology of chronic stress-related psychiatric disorders: evidence from molecular imaging studies." *Chronic Stress* 1 (2017):10.1177/2470547017710916.

216. Kennedy, D.O. "B vitamins and the brain: mechanisms, dose and efficacy – a review." *Nutrients* 8.2 (2016):68.

217. Reynolds, E. "Vitamin B12, folic acid, and the nervous system." *The Lancet Neurology* 5.11 (2006):949–60.

218. Yano, J.M., et al. "Indigenous bacteria from the gut microbiota regulate host serotonin biosynthesis." *Cell* 161.2 (2015):264–76.

219. Henderson, L., Gregory, J., Swan, G. "The National Diet and Nutrition Survey: Adults aged 19 to 64 years." Types and Quantities of Foods Consumed 1 (2002).

220. CDC. Second National Report on Biochemical Indicators of Diet and Nutrition in the US Population; US Department of Health and Human Services, Centers for Disease Control and Prevention: Hyattsville, MD, USA, 2012.

221. Morris, M.S., Jacques, P.F., Rosenberg, I.H., Selhub, J. "Folate and vitamin B-12 status in relation to anemia, macrocytosis, and cognitive impairment in older Americans in the age of folic acid fortification." *The American Journal of Clinical Nutrition* 85 (2007):193–200.

222. Wilkinson, T.J., Hanger, H.C., Elmslie, J., George, P.M., Sainsbury, R. "The response to treatment of subclinical thiamine deficiency in the elderly." *The American Journal of Clinical Nutrition* 66 (1997):925–8.

223. Sinigaglia-Coimbra, R., Lopes, A.C., Coimbra, C.G. "Riboflavin deficiency, brain function, and health." *Handbook of Behavior, Food and Nutrition*. Springer New York, 2011. pp 2427–49.

224. McGinnis, M.J., et al. "National Institutes of Health State-of-the-Science Conference Statement: multivitamin/mineral supplements and chronic disease prevention." *The American Journal of Clinical Nutrition* 85.1 (2007):257S–64S.

225. Yetley, E.A. "Multivitamin and multimineral dietary supplements: definitions, characterization, bioavailability, and drug interactions." *The American Journal of Clinical Nutrition* 85 (2007):269S–76S.

226. NIH State-of-the-Science Panel. "National Institutes of Health state-of-the-science conference statement: multivitamin/mineral supplements and chronic disease prevention." *The American Journal of Clinical Nutrition* 85 (2007):257S–64S.

227. Bailey, R.L., Gahche, J.J., Lentino, C.V., Dwyer, J.T., Engel, J.S., Thomas, P.R., et al. "Dietary supplement use in the United States: 2003–2006." *Journal of Nutrition* 141.2 (2011):261–6.

228. https://ods.od.nih.gov/factsheets/list-VitaminsMinerals/

229. Bronstein, A.C., Spyker, D.A., Cantilena, L.R. Jr, Green, J.L., Rumack, B.H., Giffin, S.L. 2008 Annual Report of the American Association of Poison Control Centers' National Poison Data System (NPDS): 26th annual report. *Clinical Toxicology* 47.10 (2009):911–1084.

230. Kennedy, D.O. "B vitamins and the brain: mechanisms, dose and efficacy – a review." *Nutrients* 8.2 (2016):68.

231. Institute of Medicine (US) Standing Committee on the Scientific Evaluation of Dietary

Reference Intakes. "Dietary reference intakes for thiamin, riboflavin, niacin, vitamin B6, folate, vitamin B12, pantothenic acid, biotin, and choline." National Academies Press (US), 1998.

232. Selhub, J., et al. "Folate-vitamin B-12 interaction in relation to cognitive impairment, anemia, and biochemical indicators of vitamin B-12 deficiency." *The American Journal of Clinical Nutrition* 89.2 (2009):702S–6S.

233. Thakkar, R.B., et al. "Acetylsalicylic acid reduces niacin extended-release-induced flushing in patients with dyslipidemia." *American Journal of Cardiovascular Drugs* 9.2 (2009):69–79.

234. Ebbing, M., et al. "Cancer incidence and mortality after treatment with folic acid and vitamin ` B12." *Jama* 302.19 (2009):2119–26.

235. Brasky, T.M., White, E., Chen, C. "Long-term, supplemental, one-carbon metabolism-related vitamin B use in relation to lung cancer risk in the Vitamins and Lifestyle (VITAL) Cohort. *Journal of Clinical Oncology* 35.30 (2017):3440–8.

236. Panossian, A., et al. "Synergy and antagonism of active constituents of ADAPT-232 on transcriptional level of metabolic regulation of isolated neuroglial cells." *Frontiers in Neuroscience* 7 (2013):16.

237. Panossian, A. "Understanding adaptogenic activity: specificity of the pharmacological action of adaptogens and other phytochemicals." *Annals of the New York Academy of Sciences* 1401.1 (2017):49–64.

238. Panossian, A., Wikman, G. "Effects of adaptogens on the central nervous system and the molecular mechanisms associated with their stress – protective activity." *Pharmaceuticals* 3.1 (2010):188–224.

239. Panossian, A., Wikman, G., Sarris, J. "Rosenroot (Rhodiola rosea): traditional use, chemical composition, pharmacology and clinical efficacy. *Phytomedicine* 17.7 (2010):481–93.

240. Hovhannisyan, A., Nylander, M., Wikman, G., Panossian, A. "Efficacy of adaptogenic supplements on adapting to stress: a randomized, controlled trial." *Journal of Athletic Enhancement* 4.4 (2015).

241. Ahmed, M. et al. "Rhodiola rosea exerts antiviral activity in athletes following a competitive marathon race." *Frontiers in Nutrition* 2 (2015):24. PMC. Web. 3 Nov. 2017.

242. Powers, S.K., Jackson, M.J. "Exercise-induced oxidative stress: cellular mechanisms and impact on muscle force production." *Physiological Reviews* 88.4 (2008):1243–76.

243. Olsson, E.M.G., von Schéele, B., Panossian, A.G. "A randomised, double-blind, placebo-controlled, parallel-group study of the standardised extract shr-5 of the roots of Rhodiola rosea in the treatment of subjects with stress-related fatigue." *Planta Medica* 75.2 (2009):105–12.

244. Edwards, D., Heufelder, A., Zimmermann, A. "Therapeutic effects and safety of Rhodiola rosea extract WS* 1375 in subjects with life–stress symptoms – results of an open–label study." *Phytotherapy Research* 26.8 (2012):1220–5.

245. Yu, S., et al. "Neuroprotective effects of salidroside in the PC12 cell model exposed to hypoglycemia and serum limitation." *Cellular and Molecular Neurobiology* 28.8 (2008):1067–78.

246. Van Diermen, D., et al. "Monoamine oxidase inhibition by Rhodiola rosea L. roots." *Journal of Ethnopharmacology* 122.2 (2009):397–401.

247. Hung, S.K., Perry, R., and Ernst, E. "The effectiveness and efficacy of Rhodiola rosea L.: a systematic review of randomized clinical trials." *Phytomedicine* 18.4 (2011):235–44.

248. Booker, A., et al. "The authenticity and quality of Rhodiola rosea products." *Phytomedicine* 23.7 (2016):754–62.

249. Chandrasekhar, K., Kapoor, J., Anishetty, S. "A prospective, randomized double-blind, placebo-controlled study of safety and efficacy of a high-concentration full-spectrum extract of ashwagandha root in reducing stress and anxiety in adults." *Indian Journal of Psychological Medicine* 34.3 (2012):255–62. PMC. Web. 12 Nov. 2017.

250. Choudhary, D., Bhattacharyya, S., Joshi, K. "Body weight management in adults under chronic stress through treatment with ashwagandha root extract: a double-blind, randomized, placebo-controlled trial." *Journal of Evidence-Based Complementary and Alternative Medicine* 22.1 (2017):96–106.

251. Bhatnagar, M., Sharma, D., Salvi, M. "Neuroprotective effects of Withania somnifera dunal: a possible mechanism." *Neurochemical Research* 34.11 (2009):1975–83.

252. Kuboyama, T., Tohd, C., and Komatsu, K. "Effects of Ashwagandha (roots of Withania somnifera) on neurodegenerative diseases." *Biological and Pharmaceutical Bulletin* 37.6 (2014):892–7.

253. Kumar, P., Kuma, A. "Possible neuroprotective effect of Withania somnifera root extract against 3-nitropropionic acid-induced behavioral, biochemical, and mitochondrial dysfunction in an animal model of Huntington's disease." *Journal of Medicinal Food* 12.3 (2009):591–600.

254. Prakash, J., et al. "Neuroprotective role of Withania somnifera root extract in Maneb-Paraquat induced mouse model of Parkinsonism." *Neurochemical Research* 38.5 (2013):972–80.

255. Kumar, A., Harikesh, K. "Protective effect of Withania somnifera Dunal on the behavioral and biochemical alterations in sleep-disturbed mice (Grid over water suspended method)." *Indian Journal of Experimental Biology* 45.6 (2007):524–8.

256. Kumar, A., Kalonia, H. "Effect of Withania somnifera on sleep-wake cycle in sleep-disturbed rats: possible GABAergic mechanism." *Indian Journal of Pharmaceutical Sciences* 70.6 (2008):806–10.

257. Morgan, A., Stevens, J. "Does Bacopa monnieri improve memory performance in older persons? Results of a randomized, placebo-controlled, double-blind trial." *The Journal of Alternative and Complementary Medicine* 16.7 (2010):753–9.

258. Finsterwald, C., Alberini, C.M. "Stress and glucocorticoid receptor-dependent mechanisms in long-term memory: from adaptive responses to psychopathologies." *Neurobiology of Learning and Memory* 112 (2014):17–29. PMC. Web. 5 December 2017.

259. Kumar, N., et al. "Efficacy of standardized extract of Bacopa monnieri (Bacognize®) on cognitive functions of medical students: a six-week, randomized placebo-controlled trial." *Journal of Evidence-Based Complementary and Alternative Medicine* 2016 (2016).

260. Kean, D., Downey, L.A., Stough, C. "A systematic review of the Ayurvedic medicinal herb Bacopa monnieri in child and adolescent populations." *Complementary Therapies in Medicine* 29 (2016):56–62.

261. Rai, D., et al. "Adaptogenic effect of Bacopa monniera (Brahmi)." *Pharmacology, Biochemistry and Behavior* 75.4 (2003):823–30.

262. Bhaskar, M., Jagtap, A.G. "Exploring the possible mechanisms of action behind the

antinociceptive activity of Bacopa monniera." *International Journal of Ayurveda Research* 2.1 (2011):2–7.

263. Rauf, K., et al. "Preclinical profile of bacopasides from Bacopa monnieri (BM) as an emerging class of therapeutics for management of chronic pains." *Current Medicinal Chemistry* 20.8 (2013):1028–37.

264. Arab, L., Liu, W., Elashoff, D. "Green and black tea consumption and risk of stroke." *Stroke* 40.5 (2009):1786–92.

265. Alexopoulos, N., et al. "The acute effect of green tea consumption on endothelial function in healthy individuals." *European Journal of Cardiovascular Prevention and Rehabilitation* 15.3 (2008):300–5.

266. Chen, X., et al. "Preventive effects of catechins on cardiovascular disease." *Molecules* 21.12 (2016):1759.

267. Ras, R.T., Zock, P.L., Draijer, R. "Tea consumption enhances endothelial-dependent vasodilation; a meta-analysis." *PLOS ONE* 6.3 (2011):e16974

268. Lorenz, M., et al. "A constituent of green tea, epigallocatechin-3-gallate, activates endothelial nitric oxide synthase by a phosphatidylinositol-3-OH-kinase-, cAMP-dependent protein kinase-, and Akt-dependent pathway and leads to endothelial-dependent vasorelaxation." *Journal of Biological Chemistry* 279.7 (2004):6190–5.

269. Adhikary, R., Mandal, V. "L-theanine: A potential multifaceted natural bioactive amide as health supplement." *Asian Pacific Journal of Tropical Biomedicine* 7.9 (2017):842–8.

270. Egashira, N., Hayakawa, K., Osajima, M., Mishima, K., Iwasaki, K., Oishi, R., Fujiwara, M. "Involvement of GABA(A) receptors in the neuroprotective effect of theanine on focal cerebral ischemia in mice." *Journal of Pharmacological Sciences* 105.2 (2007):211–4.

271. Owen, G.N., et al. "The combined effects of L-theanine and caffeine on cognitive performance and mood." *Nutritional Neuroscience* 11.4 (2008):193–8.

272. Yokogoshi, H., et al. "Effect of theanine, r-glutamylethylamide, on brain monoamines and striatal dopamine release in conscious rats." *Neurochemical Research* 23.5 (1998):667–73.

273. Song, C.H., Jung, J.H., Oh, J.S., Kim, K.S. "Effects of theanine on the release of alpha brain waves in adult males." *Korean Journal of Nutrition* 36 (2003):918–23.

274. Juneja, L.R., Chu, D., Okubo, T., Nagato, Y., Yokogoshi, H. "L-theanine – a unique amino acid of green tea and its relaxation effects in humans." *Trends in Food Science and Technology* 10.6–7 (1999):199–204.

275. Kimura, K., et al. "L-Theanine reduces psychological and physiological stress responses." *Biological Psychology* 74.1 (2007):39–45.

276. Takeda, A., et al. "Unique induction of CA1 LTP components after intake of theanine, an amino acid in tea leaves and its effect on stress response." *Cellular and Molecular Neurobiology* 32.1 (2012):41–8.

277. Tian, Xia, et al. "Protective effect of l-theanine on chronic restraint stress-induced cognitive impairments in mice." *Brain Research* 1503 (2013):24–32.

277a. Bruce, S.E., et al. "Improvements in concentration, working memory and sustained attention following consumption of a natural citicoline-caffeine beverage." *International Journal of Food Sciences and Nutrition* 65.8 (2014):1003–7.

278. Beaven, M.C., et al. "Dose effect of caffeine on testosterone and cortisol responses to resistance exercise." *International Journal of Sport Nutrition and Exercise Metabolism* 18.2 (2008):131–41.

279. Keijzers, G.B., et al. "Caffeine can decrease insulin sensitivity in humans." *Diabetes Care* 25.2 (2002):364–9.

280. Alzoubi, K.H., et al. "Caffeine prevents cognitive impairment induced by chronic psychosocial stress and/or high fat-high carbohydrate diet." *Behavioural Brain Research* 237 (2013):7–14.

281. Crozier, S.J., et al. "Cacao seeds are a 'Super Fruit': a comparative analysis of various fruit powders and products." *Chemistry Central Journal* 5.1 (2011):5.

282. Society of Chemical Industry. "Cocoa 'vitamin' health benefits could outshine penicillin." *ScienceDaily*, 12 March 2007. www.sciencedaily.com/releases/2007/03/070311202024. htm.

283. Hollenberg, N.K., Fisher, N.D.L., McCullough, M.L. "Flavanols, the Kuna, cocoa consumption, and nitric oxide." *Journal of the American Society of Hypertension* 3.2 (2009):105–12.

284. Kawabata, K., Kawai, Y., Terao, J. "Suppressive effect of quercetin on acute stress-induced hypothalamic-pituitary-adrenal axis response in Wistar rats." *The Journal of Nutritional Biochemistry* 21.5 (2010):374–80.

285. Haleagrahara, N., et al. "Flavonoid quercetin protects against swimming stress-induced changes in oxidative biomarkers in the hypothalamus of rats." *European Journal of Pharmacology* 621.1 (2009):46–52.

286. Wirtz, P.H., et al. "Dark chocolate intake buffers stress reactivity in humans." *Journal of the American College of Cardiology* 63.21 (2014):2297–9.

287. Kuebler, U., et al. "Dark chocolate attenuates intracellular pro-inflammatory reactivity to acute psychosocial stress in men: a randomized controlled trial." *Brain, Behavior, and Immunity* 57 (2016):200–8.

288. Mitchell, E.S., Slettenaar, M., van der Meer, N., Transler, C., Jans, L., Quadt, F., et al. "Differential contributions of theobromine and caffeine on mood, psychomotor performance and blood pressure." *Physiology & Behavior*, 104 (2011):816e822.

289. Scholey, A.B., French, S.J., Morris, P.J., Kennedy, D.O., Milne, A.L., & Haskell, C.F. "Consumption of cocoa flavanols results in acute improvements in mood and cognitive performance during sustained mental effort." *Journal of Psychopharmacology*, 24.10 (2010):1505–14.

290. Mastroiacovo, D., Kwik-Uribe, C., Grassi, D., Necozione, S., Raffaele, A., Pistacchio, L., et al. "Cocoa flavanol consumption improves cognitive function, blood pressure control, and metabolic profile in elderly subjects: the Cocoa, Cognition, and Aging (CoCoA) Study – a randomized controlled trial." *The American Journal of Clinical Nutrition* 101.3, (2015):538–48.

291. Crichton, G.E., Elias, M.F., Alkerwi, A. "Chocolate intake is associated with better cognitive function: The Maine-Syracuse Longitudinal Study." *Appetite* 100 (2016):126–32.

292. Sokolov, Alexander N., et al. "Chocolate and the brain: neurobiological impact of cocoa flavanols on cognition and behavior." *Neuroscience & Biobehavioral Reviews* 37.10 (2013):2445–53.

293. Van Praag, H., Lucero, M.J., Yeo, G.W., Stecker, K., Heivand, N., Zhao, C., Yip, E., Afanador, M., Schroeter, H., Hammerstone, J., Gage, F.H. "Plant-derived flavanol (-) epicatechin enhances angiogenesis and retention of spatial memory in mice." *Journal of Neuroscience* 27, (2007):5869–78.

294. Buijsse, B., et al. "Cocoa intake, blood pressure, and cardiovascular mortality: the Zutphen Elderly Study." *Archives of Internal Medicine* 166.4 (2006):411–7.

295. Katz, D.L., Doughty, K., Ali, A. "Cocoa and chocolate in human health and disease." *Antioxidants & Redox Signaling* 15.10 (2011):2779–811. PMC. Web. 6 June 2018.

296. Serafini, M., et al. "Plasma antioxidants from chocolate." *Nature* 424.6952 (2003):1013.

297. World Health Organization (WHO). Global Status Report on Alcohol and Health. p. XIV. 2014 ed. Available at: http://www.who.int/substance_abuse/publications/global_alcohol_report/msb_gsr_2014_1.pdf?ua=1. Accessed 1/18/17.

298. Bose, J., et al. "Key substance use and mental health indicators in the United States: results from the 2015 National Survey on Drug Use and Health." Substance Abuse and Mental Health Services Administration website. https://www. samhsa. gov/data/sites/default/ files/NSDUH-FFR1-2015/NSDUH-FFR1-2015/NSDUH-FFR1-2015.pdf. Published September (2016).

299. Ducci, F., Goldman, D. "Genetic approaches to addiction: genes and alcohol." *Addiction* 103 (2008):1414–28.

300. Cao, Y., Willett, W.C., Rimm, E.B., Stampfer, M.J., Giovannucci, E.L. "Light to moderate intake of alcohol, drinking patterns, and risk of cancer: results from two prospective US cohort studies." *BMJ* 351 (2015):h4328.

301. Topiwala, A., et al. "Moderate alcohol consumption as risk factor for adverse brain outcomes and cognitive decline: longitudinal cohort study." *BMJ* 357 (2017):j2353.

302. Mukamal, K.J., et al. "Alcohol consumption and risk of coronary heart disease in older adults: the cardiovascular health study." *Journal of the American Geriatrics Society* 54.1 (2006):30–7.

303. Costanzo, S., et al. "Alcohol consumption and mortality in patients with cardiovascular disease: a meta-analysis." *Journal of the American College of Cardiology* 55.13 (2010):1339–47.

304. Carlsson, S., Hammar, N., Grill, V. "Alcohol consumption and type 2 diabetes." *Diabetologia* 48.6 (2005):1051–4.

305. Di Castelnuovo, A., et al. "Alcohol dosing and total mortality in men and women: an updated meta-analysis of 34 prospective studies." *Archives of Internal Medicine* 166.22 (2006):2437–45.

306. Peters, R., Peters, J., Warner, J., Beckett, N., Bulpitt, C. "Alcohol, dementia and cognitive decline in the elderly: a systematic review." *Age and Ageing* 37.5 (2008):505–12. doi: 10.1093/ageing/afn095.

307. Ganguli, M., Vander Bilt, J., Saxton, J.A., Shen, C., Dodge, H.H. "Alcohol consumption and cognitive function in late life: a longitudinal community study." *Neurology* 65.8 (2005):1210–7.

308. Kesse-Guyot, E., Andreeva, V.A., Jeandel, C., et al. "Alcohol consumption in midlife and cognitive performance assessed 13 years later in the SU.VI.MAX 2 cohort." *PLOS ONE.* 7.12 (2012):e52311.

309. Downer, B., et al. "Effects of alcohol consumption on cognition and regional brain volumes among older adults." *American Journal of Alzheimer's Disease & Other Dementias* 30.4 (2015):364–74.

310. Corbin, W.R., Farmer, N.M., Nolen-Hoeksema, S. "Relations among stress, coping strategies, coping motives, alcohol consumption and related problems: a mediated moderation model." *Addictive Behaviors* 38 (2013):1912–9.

311. Rachdaoui, N., Sarkar, D.K. "Effects of alcohol on the endocrine system." *Endocrinology and Metabolism Clinics of North America* 42.3 (2013):593–615. doi:10.1016/j.ecl.2013.05.008.

312. Thayer, J.F., Hall, M., Sollers, J.J. III, et al. "Alcohol use, urinary cortisol, and heart rate variability in apparently healthy men: evidence for impaired inhibitory control of the HPA axis in heavy drinkers." *International Journal of Psychophysiology* 59.3 (2006):244–50.

313. Badrick, E., Bobak, M., Britton, A., Kirschbaum, C., Marmot, M., Kumari, M. "The relationship between alcohol consumption and cortisol secretion in an aging cohort." *Journal of Clinical Endocrinology & Metabolism* 93.3 (2008):750–7. doi:10.1210/jc.2007–0737.

314. Boschloo, L., et al. "Heavy alcohol use, rather than alcohol dependence, is associated with dysregulation of the hypothalamic-pituitary-adrenal axis and the autonomic nervous system." *Drug and Alcohol Dependence* 116.1 (2011):170–6.

315. Malarkey, W.B., et al. "Chronic stress down-regulates growth hormone gene expression in peripheral blood mononuclear cells of older adults." *Endocrine* 5.1 (1996):33–9.

316. Devesa, J., Almengló, C., Devesa, P. "Multiple effects of growth hormone in the body: is it really the hormone for growth?" *Clinical Medicine Insights: Endocrinology and Diabetes* 9 (2016):47–71.

317. Chrousos, G.P., Gold, P.W. "A healthy body in a healthy mind – and vice versa – the damaging power of 'uncontrollable' stress." *Journal of Clinical Endocrinology & Metabolism* 83.6 (1998):1842–5.

318. Valimaki, M., Tuominen, J.A., Huhtaniemi, I., et al. "The pulsatile secretion of gonadotropins and growth hormone, and the biological activity of luteinizing hormone in men acutely intoxicated with ethanol." *Alcoholism: Clinical and Experimental Research* 14 (1990):928–31.

319. Soszynski, P.A., Frohman, L.A. "Inhibitory effects of ethanol on the growth hormone (GH)-releasing hormone-GH-insulin-like growth factor-I axis in the rat." *Endocrinology* 131 (1992):2603–8.

320. Jimenez, V., Cardinali, D.P., Cano, P., et al. "Effect of ethanol on 24-hour hormonal changes in peripubertal male rats." *Alcohol* 34 (2004):127–32.

321. Taren, A.A., Creswell, D.J., Gianaros, P.J. "Dispositional mindfulness co-varies with smaller amygdala and caudate volumes in community adults." *PLOS ONE* 8.5 (2013):e64574.